Outpatient Invasive Radiologic Procedures

Diagnostic and Therapeutic

ARTHUR B. DUBLIN, M.D.

Associate Professor of Diagnostic Radiology
University of California, Davis
School of Medicine
Sacramento, California

1989
W. B. SAUNDERS COMPANY
Harcourt Brace Jovanovich, Inc.
Philadelphia • London • Toronto • Montreal • Sydney • Tokyo

W. B. SAUNDERS COMPANY
Harcourt Brace Jovanovich, Inc.

The Curtis Center
Independence Square West
Philadelphia, PA 19106

Library of Congress Cataloging-in-Publication Data

Outpatient invasive radiologic procedures.

Includes index.

1. Diagnostic imaging.   2. Radiology, Interventional.
   3. Ambulatory medical care.   I. Dublin, Arthur Brooks.
   [DNLM: 1. Radiography.   2. Radiotherapy. WN 200 094]

RC78.7.D53087 1989   616.07'57   88-34894

ISBN 0–7216–1532–5

Editor: Lisette Bralow
Designer: Bill Donnelly
Production Manager: Bill Preston
Manuscript Editor: Wendy Andresen
Cover Designer: Joanne Carroll
Indexer: Ella Shapiro

Outpatient Invasive Radiologic
Procedures: Diagnostic and Therapeutic   ISBN 0–7216–1532–5

Last digit is the print number: 9   8   7   6   5   4   3   2   1

To my wife, Kathryn Grant Dublin, to my sons, Matt and Jim, and to my father, William B. Dublin, M.A., M.D.

Contributors

Stanley P. Fleshman, B.A., J.D., ESQ. ■ Associate, Freidberg Law Corporation, Sacramento, California ■ *Malpractice in Diagnostic Radiology; Patients Are Not the Only Ones Exposed*

Karen K. Lindfors, M.D. ■ Assistant Professor, Division of Diagnostic Radiology, Department of Radiology, University of California, Davis, School of Medicine; Chief of Mammography, University of California, Davis, Medical Center, Sacramento, California ■ *Interventional Procedures for the Breast*

Daniel B. Kopans, M.D. ■ Associate Professor of Radiology, Harvard Medical School; Director of Breast Imaging, Massachusetts General Hospital, Boston, Massachusetts ■ *Interventional Procedures for the Breast*

John P. McGahan, M.D. ■ Professor of Radiology, University of California, Davis, School of Medicine; Chief, Section of Ultrasound, Department of Radiology, University of California, Davis, Medical Center, Sacramento, California ■ *Ultrasonographic Aspiration and Biopsy Techniques*

Frederick Hanson, M.D. ■ Professor of Obstetrics and Gynecology, University of California, Davis, School of Medicine, Sacramento, California ■ *Ultrasonographic Aspiration and Biopsy Techniques*

David C. Dwyer, M.D. ■ Staff Radiologist, Swedish Hospital Medical Center, Seattle, Washington ■ *Outpatient Arteriography: Visceral and Peripheral Studies; Outpatient CT-Guided Percutaneous Needle Biopsy Techniques*

Hugo G. Bogren, M.D. ■ Professor of Radiology and Internal Medicine (Cardiology) and Chief of Cardiothoracic Radiology, University of California, Davis, Medical Center, Sacramento, California ■ *Digital Subtraction Angiography of the Heart and the Thoracic Vessels*

Preface

There are many reasons why outpatient diagnostic centers have become increasingly popular in the past few years, including accelerating medical costs and tightening governmental control of medicine. Not all patients are candidates for outpatient invasive procedures, but many individuals can benefit from such techniques.

This text does not include all possible invasive techniques, but it does provide much practical data from authors with firsthand experience at outpatient centers. This work will provide a framework for those wishing to establish an outpatient practice and will stimulate thought about the development and acceptance of newer techniques. In addition, we hope to demonstrate that outpatient centers can provide a safe and cost-effective environment for a variety of invasive examinations. Finally, since malpractice actions are of increasing importance to the radiologist, a brief chapter addressing some of these problems is presented.

Acknowledgments

Many individuals have contributed to this effort. I particularly wish to thank the contributing authors for their time and work on their individual chapters. Cindy McCray, Nancy Steers, and Kathryn Dublin were also helpful in the preparation of this manuscript. Finally, I wish to thank Suzanne Boyd, Deane Manke, and Dana Dreibelbis, formerly of W. B. Saunders, who helped in the inception of this work, and Lisette Bralow, Bill Preston, Peter Clifford, Wendy Andresen, Ella Shapiro, and Kate Leven, currently with W. B. Saunders in Philadelphia, for their invaluable help and support.

Contents

Planning an Outpatient Diagnostic Imaging Center

Arthur B. Dublin, M.D.

Outpatient invasive procedures can be time-consuming and exhausting, especially if the cases are complicated. However, outpatient techniques, if properly planned and managed, can be rewarding professionally and can be successful financially. Financial success not only is achieved from the procedures themselves, but also from the spin-off to other noninvasive examinations provided by an imaging center. Therefore, invasive procedures, although they may stand by themselves as a financial entity, should be thought of as part of a complete service facility. Although radiology services account for only 3 to 5% of the total yearly increase in national health care costs (the latter 6.6% as of May, 1988), these procedures have been particularly hard-hit by new federal medical policies, especially in hospital-based settings.[1-2] Some authors predict that 2,000 or more outpatient diagnostic centers will be operating by the mid 1990s, spurred on in part by the Medicare reimbursement policies (diagnosis-related groups [DRGs]).[3] Invasive procedures will be a viable part of this expansion process. This chapter will deal with the basic planning of a complete outpatient radiologic diagnostic center (using our center as a guide) and will outline the financing, management, and technical aspects of such a successful project.

THE BUSINESS PLAN

A successful imaging center needs a business plan in order to obtain initial financing, to organize the principals' goals and objectives, to allow an assessment of clinical referral patterns, and to attract an appropriate number of patients.[4] Radiologists' attempts to change established referral patterns are hampered by the following factors: (1) the loyalty of the community clinicians to established radiological practices (which may be your own former practice); (2) the loyalty of the clinicians' front office staff to the office staff of other imaging groups (very important!); (3) the general inertia—that is, the lack of a desire to change established referral patterns; and finally (4) an ignorance of new imaging techniques that are being introduced. A business plan can introduce clinicians to newer techniques, as well as to new ways of implementing established techniques (e.g., angiography in an outpatient setting). Different plans may need to be developed. For instance, a synopsis with basic data and appropriate illustrations of the proposed center may be helpful to present to prospective limited partners and referring physicians. In addition, a more comprehensive plan is needed to provide detailed financial projections and is generally useful for a presentation to large lending institutions. The following discussion is a suggested outline that might be used to construct such a detailed plan. Many of these sections overlap in order to provide a cohesiveness to the overall project.

Introduction

This part of the plan might include general statements such as the following: Hospital costs account for 37% of the health care dollar; therefore, anything that can reduce such overhead expenses is a valuable asset to the medical community. Furthermore, the DRGs implemented by Medicare do not apply to outpatient settings.[1] Thus, quality care at reasonable prices can be provided for these groups with reduced overhead costs. An overview of the scope of the imaging center, its relationship to the medical community, and a general introduction to the costs of establishing such a center should be outlined. This discussion naturally leads into the next component of a successful business plan.

Need for an Imaging Center

Many factors account for the failure of an imaging center, including poor planning, poor operational techniques, and excessive competition.[3] A facility may fail simply because the basic question "Does my community really need an imaging center?" has not been addressed and answered in a sensible fashion. There are many ways to determine such a need.[5] Polling potential limited investors is not the way to ascertain such a need, since limited partners tend to be overly optimistic regarding the numbers of patients they can send to an imaging center. Therefore, a more likely starting point is a survey of uninterested parties, especially physicians who are not likely to be investors, as well as clinicians whose loyalties may reside with other imaging groups or with inpatient facilities.[5] In addition, the need should be based on surveys of existing inpatient and outpatient facilities and of current and projected patient growth patterns. After this basic assessment, a more sophisticated analysis using the worst/ best case method is appropriate. This method allows one to look at any project from three basic vantage points: (1) the worst case (i.e., barely making a profit, if at all); (2) the most likely case, considering the projected number of patients, costs, and so on; and finally (3) the best case (assuming profits exceed predicted goals, without unanticipated costs). All of these data should be tabulated in numeric form and presented as in Table 1–1.

As mentioned above, a survey of established practices with similar technologies and patient bases is an appropriate starting point to determine the need for an imaging center. For example, a relatively small patient population could conceivably support a magnetic resonance imaging (MRI) scanner or digital angiographic room, regardless of physician investment, if no other competition were present or expected and the center were isolated geographically. On the other hand, a larger population base may actually produce a more competitive situation for a center because of increased numbers of radiologists (and thus increased price competition), increased political considerations, and increased choices of centers to which physicians, especially noninvestors, may refer their patients. Thus, personal relationships and limited partnerships will play a larger role if the facility is located in New York or Los Angeles rather than in a small isolated rural setting.

Knowledge of the attitudes of a local medical community is very important. For example, outpatient invasive procedures may not be accepted by uninformed local clinicians, and this type of radiology practice, although having many obvious advantages, thus may fail from an informational standpoint. Introductory seminars using local radiologists as well as nationally recognized experts in the field of outpatient techniques are useful in such instances. Simple newsletters and brochures can be used effectively in spreading the word to enlarge the referral base.

Inappropriate inclusion of imaging techniques may be damaging to your reputation, as well as financially ruinous. For example, an outpatient cardiac catheterization laboratory is not a wise choice if cardiology and cardiac surgery are poorly represented specialties in the local community. Thus, the proper assessment of the local medical community for newer techniques is a necessary prerequisite for success.

Description of the Principals

This section is extremely important if the radiologists are new to a community. In general, centers started by unknown physicians rarely do

Table 1–1
MOST LIKELY CASE EXAMPLE

Year	Revenue/year—Most likely case					
	1	*2*	*3*	*4*	*5*	*Total*
Mammography	458000	525000	551250	578813	607753	2720816
Ultrasonography	403040	462000	485100	509355	534823	2394318
CT	1259500	1443750	1515938	1591734	1671321	7482243
Digital angiography	291200	735000	771750	810338	850854	3459142
MRI	873600	2205000	2315250	2431013	2552563	10377426
General radiology	227626	260925	273971	287670	302053	1352245
Total	3512966	5631675	5913259	6208922	6519368	27786189

Year	Expenses/year—Most likely case					
	1	*2*	*3*	*4*	*5*	*Total*
Building lease	84000	88200	92610	97241	102103	464153
Equipment lease	0	704906	1094690	1094690	1094690	3988976
Equipment service	0	26412	41000	209720	209720	486852
Equipment insurance	5040	5292	5557	5834	6126	27849
Utilities	23400	32760	34398	36118	37924	164600
Office manager	32400	34020	35721	37507	39382	179030
P/T clerk	6300	13230	13892	14586	15315	63323
Office supplies	9000	9450	9923	10419	10940	49731
Office equipment lease	3600	3780	3969	4167	4376	19892
Examination expense	375186	560175	588184	617593	648473	2789610
Cryogens	12000	25200	26460	27783	29172	120615
Legal/accountant-fees	9000	7500	7875	8269	8682	41326
Start-up loan	230000	0	0	0	0	230000
Miscellaneous	5040	5292	5557	5834	6126	27849
Radiologist (2)	120000	180000	200000	200000	200000	900000
Malpractice insurance	12000	12600	13230	13892	14586	66308
Total	926966	1708817	2173064	2383653	2427615	9620114
Gross income	2586000	3922858	3740195	3825269	4091753	18166075

Year	Cash flow/year—Most likely case					
	1	*2*	*3*	*4*	*5*	*Total*
Start-up load	200000					
Discounted revenue	1637114	4173876	4373700	4601254	4831317	19617260
Less expenses	926966	1708817	2173064	2383653	2427615	9620114
Cash balance	910148	3375206	5575842	7793444	10197146	10197146

well unless supported by established, leading members of the local medical community. A brief outline of the background and qualifications of the imaging specialists (radiologists) should be given. Reference to and inclusion of a curriculum vitae is appropriate, and as suggested above, supporting letters from local, well-known physicians are helpful.

Scope of Services to be Offered

A brief survey of the various imaging modalities is essential and is best couched in layman's terms to be appreciated and comprehended by financial institutions and uninformed clinicians alike. A comparison with existing facilities is important, stressing the advantages of outpatient techniques.

General and Specific Geographic Demographics Pertaining to an Imaging Center

The access and convenience of an imaging center to patients should be stressed in this section.[3] Various maps of the general patient capture area (noting the proximity of your center to the location of major medical facilities and other imaging centers), a detailed map of the proposed site for the center, a modified blueprint map of the center itself (Fig. 1–1), and demographic data (broken into distant and local distributions in relationship to the outpatient facility) should be included in the plan. A more detailed discussion of the layout of an outpatient diagnostic center will be discussed in greater detail later in this chapter.

Demographic data should be broken down into age-groups, male/ female ratios (important, for instance, for projecting mammographic or prostate ultrasonic data), general population groupings by zip code or county boundaries, growth rates over the past 10 years, and projections for the future 5 years. All of these data can be obtained or extracted from local chambers of commerce, information centers, United States Census Bureau figures, and finally from professional demographic projection firms (the latter generally are not needed if one is willing to spend a modest amount of time in coordinating the statistical data).

Market Analysis

A market analysis should divide the center into each special imaging modality (e.g., mammography, digital radiography, computed tomography [CT]). Using local demographic data, realistic projections of the

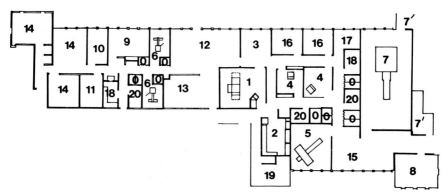

Figure 1–1. Floor plan of an outpatient imaging center. **0**: Patient changing rooms. **1**: Digital angiography, general fluoroscopy. **2**: Reading room (with DSA, CT consoles). **3**: Three-bed recovery suite. **4**: Ultrasonography. **5**: Computed tomography. **6**: Mammography. **7**: Magnetic resonance imaging (MRI). **7′**: Support equipment for MRI, including cryogenerator. **8**: Computer facility for MRI, CT, DSA. **9**: Expansion area for second fluoroscopy unit or CT. **10**: Control room for room number 9. Temporary office for chief technologist and patient coordinator. **11**: Teaching file for MRI fellows. **12**: Patient waiting room. **13**: Patient reception/checkout desk. **14**: Typing, business computers, business manager. **15**: Ancillary waiting area for CT/MRI, which also can function as an after-hours meeting area/classroom. **16**: Radiologists' offices. **17**: Technologists' lounge. **18**: Darkrooms. **19**: Plain film/tomographic room. **20**: Restrooms.

number of studies that could be done by the facility should be undertaken, with reference to different strengths or weaknesses in the specialty and subspecialty clinical groups available in the population capture area.

General Financial Analysis

Each area of the imaging center is broken down into separate cost centers, with detailed fixed and variable costs projected for each year for 5 years. A 250-day year is typically used for calculation purposes. It is extremely important to show that each element of an imaging center can be profitable on its own, although in practical terms the separate cost centers are interrelated. Table 1–2 lists the typical expenditures one might expect to encounter for each modality. As can be seen from this table, charges can be decreased if patient volume is adequately increased, with preservation of total profits. This fact is a key to any business endeavor—that is, you should concentrate on increasing (within reason, considering quality and patient comfort) the number of cases to maintain the price per unit as low as possible. Examples of projected worst case, most likely case, and best case analysis are useful (Table 1–1).

The financing of the equipment can be accomplished several ways, depending on the philosophy and expected cash flow of each center.

Table 1–2
TOTAL BREAK-EVEN PATIENT CHARGE ($)
AT VARIOUS UTILIZATION RATES

Type of Examination	Number of Examinations/Day							Sacramento Community Average Charges ($)
	2	4	6	10	15	20	30	
Screening mammography	191	111	84	62	53	47	42	—
Full mammography	209	129	102	80	71	64	60	138
Ultrasonography	253	153	118	91	78	71	64	194
Computed tomography	1482	787	553	367	276	229		606
Digital angiography	1233	782	631	511				1350
Magnetic resonance imaging	3393	1724	1169	724	502	391		772
General radiography	213	131	104	82	71	64	60	94

Lease-purchase arrangements with the manufacturer are quite common. The purchase of the equipment from a single supplier has many advantages, including the following: (1) a better price break on each piece of equipment because of the overall purchase amount, (2) a greater degree of uniformity and response for the service of the equipment, (3) a more flexible purchase agreement, including possible delayed payment schedules, and (4) greater access to new technological updates. The less favorable depreciation schedules, recently passed by Congress, will also affect the mode of purchase.

Summary and Conclusions

This section should highlight the strengths of an imaging center and should also stress the important role that such a facility will play in providing cost-effective diagnostic care for the local community.

ASPECTS OF IMAGING CENTER PARTNERSHIPS—THE PROBLEM OF SELF-REFERRAL

The construction and proper execution of an imaging center business plan may eventually necessitate the involvement of limited or general partners. These partners may be referring clinicians, and therein lie questions of ethics that have been discussed at length in the literature and, more importantly, in various state legislatures.[6–10]

Relman, editor of the *New England Journal of Medicine*, states that "Ethical practitioners minimize them [conflicts of interest] by avoiding self-referral whenever possible." Medicine, according to the American

Medical Association (AMA), is a "profession, a calling, and not a business."[11] Relman further suggests that "In admitting that business deals create conflicts of interests for physicians, but arguing that they need be concerned only about arrangements that demonstrably lead to bad practice, the AMA's statements ignore the damage done to the public trust in the medical profession by even the *appearance* of conflicts of interest." Relman concludes that the "physician must avoid any personal commercial conflict of interest that might compromise the loyalty and treatment of the patient."[12]

The American College of Radiology (ACR) policy statement suggests that it is satisfactory for a radiologist to practice in imaging centers, except "in a system which offers financial rewards for patient referrals or practice patterns which are medically inappropriate."[13] Furthermore, ownership of imaging centers "may legitimately and ethically be controlled by physicians, other organizations, such as hospitals, or some combination of corporate financing and individual investor capital, unless prohibited by law."[13]

Marasco emphasized this ACR policy statement and stressed that a threefold increase in utilization has occurred in nonradiologist, clinician-performed radiology procedures.[13] He suggests that the ACR statement provides a framework for clinicians and radiologists to work together. Furthermore, Vinocour reiterates the fact that the physician oversupply has driven clinicians to perform radiology procedures and that half of all radiology examinations are performed by nonradiologists.[14] Imaging centers that provide high quality, rapid interpretation, and comfortable facilities for their patients will succeed. In addition, a multispecialty imaging center can provide a one-stop service and has a better chance of survival than a facility offering just one modality (e.g., MRI or invasive procedures).[15–16]

The state of Michigan currently prohibits the referral of patients by physicians to radiologist-run imaging centers in which the referring clinician has *any* financial interest whatsoever.[9, 17] However, there are no laws prohibiting clinician referral to imaging facilities that clinicians operate themselves.[10] Lawyers are currently barred from having nonlawyer investors—an important reason, perhaps, why lawyers are largely insulated from the price competition affecting physicians.[10] Zeeman and Elliott raise the point that clinician investment promotes radiology by radiologists, and that "joint ventures have in many communities broken the stranglehold of self-referral and reduced volume of radiologic procedures performed by primary care physicians."[10] However, clinicians continue to perform a large percentage of radiologic studies. In our experience, it appears that pressure by health maintenance organizations (HMOs) and price control efforts have affected the practice of radiology by nonradiologists more than clinician investor–imaging center relationships.

Zeman and Elliott have divided their thoughts regarding joint ventures into four basic categories: (1) **Financial.** Investors' financial returns are based on the amount of capital they have at risk, not the number of patients they refer to the center.[10] This statement is not quite true, however, since if referrals are not adequate to produce a profit from the center there will be no financial returns. Recent tax law changes have eliminated investment tax credits; therefore, the technical component is less attractive to clinician investors.[7] Losses from centers for limited or general partners *cannot* be used to offset practice or portfolio earnings. These tax changes may therefore produce pressure to lower professional fees for the radiologist in order to compensate for tax benefit decreases and to secure continued profitability for their clinician investors. Zeman and Elliott also state that in one center as many as 50% of referrals came from physicians without a financial interest in the imaging center.[10] Of course, this figure can easily be increased to 100% if no clinicians are involved as investors! (2) **Legal.** As stated above, some states such as Michigan prohibit self-referral of physicians to centers in which they have a financial interest. California law requires physicians to disclose a financial interest of $25,000 or 5% of the value of a center.[15-16] In addition, pending state and local (Los Angeles) legislation in California would make illegal any kind of clinician investor relationships.[19] (3) **Ethics.** Although the editorials of the *New England Journal of Medicine* raise serious ethical questions about self-referral, Zeman and Elliott propose that "a Board Certified radiologist performing and interpreting imaging procedures, assessing their necessity, and billing fairly for services provided is far more ethical than the unchecked self-referral that continues to flourish in many settings."[10-12] Although this latter statement is generally true, the ability to assess the necessity of any particular examination may be seriously compromised by clinician investor politics and pressures. (4) **The perception of radiology by the public and colleagues.** As the authors state, "this area is the toughest to address." It has been our experience that some clinicians, in fact a great many of our colleagues, look on clinician investor imaging centers with distrust, if not dismay. Therefore, despite the qualifications and perceived honesty of the radiologists in such a center, the public and noninvolved clinicians may rightfully view such efforts with some suspicion.

Stevens comments on the corporate practice of imaging. "To insure that nothing interferes with a doctor's loyalty to his patients, every state except Missouri and Nebraska theoretically prohibit corporations of nondoctors from employing physicians or practicing medicine." However, these laws are often ignored. Nevertheless, certain states such as California are looking at such arrangements much more closely, suggesting that joint ventures must be structured in such a manner that the physician does not work for the corporation. In addition, the nonphysician should not interfere with medical decisions, and joint ventures must clearly divide medical from administrative responsibilities.[8]

PERSONNEL

A significant expense in running an outpatient imaging center is the cost of personnel. As compared with general clinical practices, imaging personnel costs represent a much lower fraction of the total expense outlay because of a high equipment debt service. For example, our personnel costs are roughly 15% and 25% of the debt service costs of the equipment and the total departmental costs, respectively. Therefore, we have found that generous salaries and benefits help to attract the best office and technological staff. Good technologists, at least in our locale, are becoming harder and harder to obtain. We do pay overtime when appropriate, but otherwise do not pay on an hourly basis. If salaries are 10% over and above the local going rate, this means a 10% increase of a 25% overhead rate, or an addition of only 2.5% to the total expenses.

Some facilities have bonus or incentive plans to increase patient throughput. For instance, one center has an incentive system for MRI technologists in which each technologist earns an additional $10 per patient over 10 patients examined per day. This program has resulted in a 25% increase in patient throughput.[20] We do not have such an immediate incentive plan, however, fearing that speed may compromise quality. Our personnel participate in a year-end profit-sharing program that rewards many different attributes, including speed, competency, patient relationships, and relationships with other technologists and with referring physicians and ancillary personnel. This is combined with additional reinforcements such as parties for the technologists and office staff and their families, as well as frequent sincere compliments and restrained but constructive criticism. We suggest that the latter approach fosters harmony and a "family atmosphere" instead of a game-show relationship.

One key person in any imaging center is the individual we have designated as the patient coordinator. This staff person is responsible for the smooth flow of patients from the front check-in desk to the examination room, fields compliments and complaints alike from patients, and is an invaluable advisor on patient satisfaction and the general flow of business within the department. In order to provide the best possible care for our patients, we have even given our patient coordinators the responsibility to tell us, the radiologists, if they think that we are not interacting with our patients in a prompt, courteous, and effective manner. A physician with an inflated ego has no place in a successful imaging center, and we encourage all comments and criticisms.

A nurse is generally not needed for a center of our size. Postprocedure care is handled by the technologist, the patient coordinator, or the physician. Family members are encouraged to be with the patient during the recovery process, and occasionally with anxious individuals during certain examinations. Intravenous lines are started by the radiologist, and contrast and medications are administered by the technologist. It is important that the technologist and front office staff know where the radiologist is at all times, in order to provide prompt coverage and response for emergency situations. For more unstable patients transferred from hospitals, accompanied nursing care is required.

IONIC VERSUS NONIONIC CONTRAST AGENTS

One of the aspects of planning a center's financial viability is a consideration of the projected cost of contrast materials. A cost comparison of certain ionic and nonionic agents is presented in Chapter 3, on outpatient neuroradiology techniques.[21] This particular issue is highlighted here because the introduction of nonionic materials has produced a controversy regarding the cost, appropriateness, and indications for ionic versus nonionic agents.[22–23] Some authors argue for the use of nonionic agents for *all* intravenous and intraarterial studies despite the cost concerns, but with respect for patient comfort and suggested decreased general toxicity and the possible legal liabilities of using ionic materials. Another group argues for the continued use of nonionic agents for most intravenous and some intraarterial applications and suggests that the possible lowered toxic and allergic/toxic rates for nonionic materials have not been firmly established.[22–23]

In order to provide a framework for the day-to-day use of contrast materials in our facility, a survey of local private, military, and university facilities, as well as three additional geographically distant California university centers, was undertaken. The survey concluded that "routine" intravenous studies (e.g., intravenous pyelography [IVP], CT cystogram) are still performed, for the most part, with ionic materials. For patients' comfort, nonionic agents are administered for intraarterial studies (e.g., femoral runoffs) and for certain high-risk groups such as individuals with heart disease, prior contrast reactions, and so on (Table 1–3).[22] This survey will hopefully form a rational basis for the establishment of quality of care for contrast agents, as practiced in northern California, and is a reasonable compromise between those advocating either type of agent alone for all studies.

As of May, 1987, Blue Shield has agreed to reimburse radiologists for the use of nonionic contrast media, based on the manufacturer's price list.[6] In addition, California's Medicaid program (Medi-Cal) has indicated

Table 1–3
SUGGESTED INDICATIONS FOR THE USE OF NONIONIC
OR LOW-IONIC CONTRAST AGENTS

Age: Under 1 year, over 70 years of age
Previous reaction to contrast media
Asthma; severe allergy
Cardiovascular disease
Renal failure
Severe diabetes mellitus
Clinically recognized dehydration
Blood dyscrasias (e.g., sickle cell disease)
Dysproteinemia (e.g., multiple myeloma)
Myelography, especially in combination with CT
Anxious patients
Angiography of peripheral vasculature, especially femoral runoff studies, external carotids, embolization procedures

that it will cover the extra cost for nonionic media on a "by report basis" for patients with certain risk factors.[6, 14] More generous reimbursement policies for the use of these new contrast agents will undoubtedly increase radiologists' use of these new materials.

THE ARCHITECTURAL ASPECTS OF AN IMAGING CENTER

Figure 1–1 outlines the layout of our facility. Although this plan may not be ideal for every group, it does demonstrate what can be done by renovating an existing building to produce an imaging center. As pointed out by Seago, a single-floor plan has many advantages over a multiple-story site.[5] The most obvious benefits are the continuity of patient flow and a lack of dependence on elevator transport (the latter is especially important for semi- or nonambulatory individuals). In addition, although MRI units can be placed in second story or higher locations, the additional structural support and under-unit radio-frequency shielding for such elevated units can be quite expensive.

Approximately 6,400 square feet were allotted to our facility, including the business office space, bathrooms, changing areas, and storage room. The remaining 9,000 square feet of the building (mostly the second floor) are leased to a variety of physician and nonphysician groups. Figure 1–1 shows the distribution of specialty areas within the department. The MRI (Philips Medical Systems Gyroscan 1.5 tesla) is shielded by a steel dome, as well as by steel plate above and to each side of the magnet. Five-gauss field strengths are maintained just outside the MRI room. Radio-frequency protection is simplified by placing the copper mesh just outside the magnet's bore. The CT/MRI patient waiting area allows patients to observe the experience of preceding patients within the devices and to ask questions and view an introductory videotape on the two procedures. Patient preparation is expedited by the patient coordinator, a procedure that allows the technicians to devote all of their energy to the actual scanning process.

Biopsy procedures are usually performed in the CT or ultrasonography suites. Cellular material is immediately screened at the center by the cytopathologist, who helps to determine the success of the biopsy specimens. Recovery for angiography, myelography, biopsy, and hospital transfer patients is provided in a suite situated adjacent to the angiography area. A fully stocked, mobile crash cart with defibrillator is available in angiography and can be rapidly moved to any area within the department. Automatically dialed emergency numbers are preprogrammed to reach a nearby surgery center, as well as local appropriate internists and surgeons. In addition, small kits with basic antiallergic reaction medications (epinephrine, diphenhydramine, steroids) are placed in the IVP and CT suites.

The waiting area (room 12 in Fig. 1–1) also has access to an outdoor garden area behind the building, an arrangement that is especially useful for smokers or young children. The business office (room 14 in Fig. 1–1) is separated from the flow of traffic and from the mammography suites by a controlled doorway. Patients wishing to register complaints or ask questions about their bills are directed via an outside hallway to the business office entrance. All patients existing or entering the imaging facility must pass by the reception and payment desk. Room 11 (Fig. 1–1) is currently used as a teaching file for visiting MRI fellows but could be easily converted to a second radiologist's reading room.

The current reading room arrangement is ideal for rapid consultation between the radiologists and is centrally placed for reasonable access to all diagnostic areas. CT can be easily monitored via a separate physician viewing console, which also performs reformation computations. Two cameras (14 × 14-inch or 8 × 10-inch format) are designed to function from either the MRI, CT, or the physician's CT console, in order to provide backup for each unit.

Some disadvantages of this plan include (1) the degree of adaptation and compromise that results from renovating an existing building, (2) the presence of patient traffic between the angiographic suite and recovery, (3) some increased travel for the mammographic technologist to the primary reading room to have films checked, and (4) the mildly inadequate dressing room space during the hours of very heavy use of the ultrasonography area.

References

1. Steinberg EP: The impact of regulation and payment innovations on acquisition of new imaging technologies. Radiol Clin North Am 23:381–389, 1983.
2. United States Bureau of Labor Statistics, May, 1988.
3. De Wolfe A: Good marketing— a key ingredient to a successful imaging center. Diagn Imag March:137–142, 1987.
4. Fever S: Joint ventures: Why a business plan is essential. Med Econom 30:62–67, 1987.
5. Seago K: Imaging center design and construction: Good planning pays off. Appl Radiol February: 37–42, 1987.
6. Bull Am Coll Radiol 43:3, 1987.
7. Johnson RS: Shifts in health-care economics bring business focus to radiologists. Diagn Imag March:75–77, 1985.
8. Stevens C: Joint ventures: Don't let the law take you by surprise. Med Econom 30:52–61, 1987.
9. Thomas MC: Joint ventures: Who knows what evil lurks. Med Econom 30:47–51, 1987.
10. Zeman RK, Elliott LP: Physician investment in free-standing imaging centers: In defense. AJR 147:414–416, 1986.
11. Relman AS: Dealing with conflicts of interest. N Engl J Med 313:749–751, 1985.
12. Relman AS: Antitrust law and the physician entrepreneur. N Engl J Med 313:884–885, 1985.
13. Hirschtick SR, Chenen AR, Lemon BS, et al: Free-standing imaging centers. A resource monograph prepared at the request of the American College of Radiology. 1985.
14. Vinocour B: Self-referral runs head-on into radiologists' economic interests. Diagn Imag March:44–45, 1985.
15. Hess TP: Doc in the box comes to radiology. Diagn Imag March:46–52, 1985.
16. Hess TP: Skills of technologist can make or break an MRI center. Diagn Imag February:85–93, 1987.
17. Baum S: Physician investment in free-standing imaging centers: In opposition. AJR 147:412–413, 1986.
18. Huston PL: Joint ventures: Choosing the best tax strategy. Med Econom 30:68–73, 1987.
19. Moore G: Assembly bill number 1232, State of California, 1987.
20. MRI focus. The Cooperative. Del Mar, Calif, April/May, 1987.
21. Dublin AB: Outpatient angiography of the brain, head and neck. *In* Dublin AB (ed): Outpatient invasive radiologic procedures—diagnostic and therapeutic. WB Saunders, Philadelphia, 1988.
22. McClellan BL: Low-osmolality contrast media; premises and promises. Radiol Soc North Am Annu Meet (Chicago), November, 1986.
23. Hess TP: High costs make nonionics painful drugs to adopt. Appl Radiol January:117–132, 1987.
24. Ikeda R: Personal communication. June, 1987.

CHAPTER 2

Malpractice in Diagnostic Radiology; Patients Are Not the Only Ones Exposed

Stanley P. Fleshman, Esq.

Diagnostic radiologic imaging has experienced a technologic and clinical revolution in the past decade. What was once viewed as science fiction is now simply science, and what was once fiction verges on fact. As will be seen in this chapter, this technologic revolution has substantial impact not only on the practice of diagnostic radiologic imaging but also on the malpractice exposure faced in that discipline.

Before engaging in that discussion, however, there must be some reference to the theories regulating the legal liability that may be imposed on a physician. The theoretic bases of liability range from assault and battery and fraud to breach of warranty. However, the primary theories confronting the physician are, first, negligence and, second, failure to comply with the requirements of informed consent.

When a physician undertakes treatment of a patient, including performing diagnostic procedures, that physician assumes a duty imposed by law to "have that degree of learning and skill ordinarily possessed by reputable physicians practicing in the same or similar locality and under similar circumstances."[1] The physician has the additional duty "to use the care and skill ordinarily exercised in like cases by reputable members of the profession practicing in the same or similar locality under similar circumstances."[2]

When a physician is a specialist, such as a diagnostic radiologist, the standard to which he or she is held includes not only the general standards of a physician as just indicated but also the requirement that the physician have and use the knowledge, care, and skill ordinarily used by reputable specialists in the same field.[3] These duties, in essence, define the legal standard of care against which the acts of omissions by a physician will be measured by judges and juries.

The one area of evolution in these legal standards concerns the so-called locality requirement. There is great force to the proposition that in highly specialized medical disciplines, such as diagnostic radiology, there should be no locality standard, but that instead the standard should be universal in nature. This approach is the consequence of wider availability of the most recent and sophisticated equipment, the universality of board certification requirements, and the abundance of and accessibility to the latest in medical research and experience. The practitioner in a small, remote community may possess the latest equipment and, by use of a personal computer, have access to the world's medical literature, thereby imposing on himself or herself the same standard as a practitioner in a large metropolitan community. Therefore, as a practical matter, if one is engaged in the practice of diagnostic radiology, one should expect to be held to the standard of care of a physician in a big city, or possibly even of one affiliated with a university.

Under the negligence theory of liability, the patient must prove that the physician failed to meet the standard of care and that such failure was the proximate or legal cause of the injuries and damages sustained by the patient. The damages recoverable under a negligence theory are those damages that are compensatory in nature. They may include damages for pain and suffering, lost earnings or lost capacity to earn a living, and medical expenses incurred as a result of the patient's injuries. The nature and amount of such damages may vary from minuscule to monumental.

Many times the most difficult issue for the patient to prove in litigating a medical negligence case is whether the physician's acts or omissions were in fact the cause of the injuries sustained by the patient. This issue may be presented in the context of diagnostic radiology when the alleged error is the failure to diagnose the presence of a tumor. Merely proving that the physician missed the diagnosis does not ensure the patient a monetary recovery. The patient must further prove that had the diagnosis been more timely, some form of treatment of the tumor would have resulted in a cure or lengthening of the patient's life expectancy. Depending on the nature of the tumor and the clinical stage at which it is discovered and treated, this burden of proof may be impossible to meet.

The second major area of exposure to the diagnostic radiologist concerns a failure to comply with the requirements of informed consent. It has been the law for many years that a physician has a duty to the patient to disclose all material information necessary to enable the patient to make an informed decision regarding proposed operations or treatment.[4] This duty is not necessarily circumscribed by what physicians in the community disclose or withhold. The physician must instead disclose information that he or she knows, or should know, would be regarded as significant by a reasonable person in deciding to accept or reject a recommended medical procedure. For example, if the procedure involves a risk of death or serious bodily harm, the physician must disclose such possibilities in layman's terms and disclose the complications that might arise from the proposed procedure.

Of particular significance to the diagnostic radiologist is the duty of a physician to disclose all material information to a patient to enable the patient to make an informed decision regarding whether to take or refuse a diagnostic test. This disclosure includes informing the patient of the risk incurred if the test is refused.[5] Thus, in theory, the diagnostic radiologist must disclose to the patient the risk of death or serious disability inherent in procedures to be performed and the risks confronting the patient if a recommended procedure is refused. In practice, of course, the patient is most likely to be advised of these matters by the referring physician, so that by merely appearing at the radiology center the patient may evidence an understanding of the need for the procedure.

Failure to comply with the requirements of informed consent exposes the physician to liability for any injury and damage resulting from the procedure if the jury finds that a reasonably prudent person would not have undergone the procedure had the risks been adequately explained. This liability is not conditional on whether or not the procedure was properly performed.

Although the theories of liability have changed little in recent years, the implementation of those theories has undergone some considerable restructuring. In California, for example, the legislature perceived there to be a medical malpractice crisis in the mid-1970s, and as a consequence of that perception, a body of legislation was enacted to deal specifically with medical malpractice claims. That legislation restricted the amount of financial recovery for pain and suffering damages, restricted attorneys' fees payable to the patients' attorneys, and substantially affected various other aspects of malpractice litigation. After years of litigation in the appellate courts, this legislation was finally held to be constitutional. Courts in other states, however, have held similar legislation not to be constitutional.

As part of the legislation viewed to be protective of physicians, there have been imposed requirements that a Certificate of Merit be filed by the patient's attorney, certifying that after review by an appropriate physician the attorney believes there is probable cause to bring the claim. Although this requirement may have had some dampening effect on otherwise unmeritorious lawsuits, it has had the ironic side effect of substantially eliminating physicians' claims for malicious prosecution against plaintiffs' attorneys who pursue cases that are truly unmeritorious. Physicians are often eager to sue those who prosecute them; however, courts have viewed the Certificate of Merit as providing an attorney with probable cause for instituting a medical malpractice case and, thus, insulating him or her from liability for maliciously prosecuting that case.

A more recent modification of the tort system, intended to be at least palliative of its perceived abuse, may have unintended side effects. In California, the electorate passed Proposition 51, which sought to alter the theory of joint and several liability, such as to restrict a defendant's obligation to pay certain types of damages to that defendant's percentage of liability for the injury. Thus, where previously a joint wrongdoer may have been required to pay 100% of the damages although he was only 50% at fault, Proposition 51 now restricts that defendant's payment solely to his 50% of the damages. This change, however, creates greater uncertainty for the plaintiff in terms of from whom he or she will be able to recover the entirety of the damages sustained. To help assuage this uncertainty, the plaintiff now is inclined to join any and all physicians who participated in the care and treatment of the injured patient, rather than solely those who were primarily responsible. The potential result, therefore, is that more physicians may be dragged into litigation when they were only marginally involved in the patient's care and treatment. Moreover, there may now be more incentive for physicians to blame each other, rather than present the traditional united defense. The ultimate impact of laws such as Proposition 51 on the exposure of the physician to litigation is still to be determined.

How the traditional theories of liability interact with the changing practice of diagnostic radiology is also still to be determined. However, the following are some observations that may be of interest. In addition to the technologic strides taken in the practice of diagnostic radiology, there has been a social, economic, and clinical revolution in that practice. In the past, the radiologist practiced primarily in association with a hospital facility that most likely was the only repository of the latest sophisticated equipment. Such physicians may now practice in outpatient facilities physically detached from major hospitals. Such circumstances may have substantial impact on the exposure to malpractice claims.

In large part, an outpatient center's economic existence depends on establishing a referral base from both private physicians and institutions. However, the radiologist may be placed in a position of questioning the need for the prescribed procedures, the extent to which the procedure should be done, the benefits of a procedure versus the risks inherent therein, and other matters with regard to the workup by the referring physician or facility. Although the physician's duty to the patient may require such questions, the center's economic well-being may sometimes be difficult to ignore, given the substantial investment that new technology requires. On the other hand, the law imposes on the radiologist the duties previously discussed, and the failure to meet those duties may result in lawsuits that are surely a more significant economic burden than the loss of some referrals.

From a medical malpractice perspective, the increasing technology in the practice of diagnostic radiology has spawned both benefit and burden. The benefits include the possibility that fewer invasive procedures, which may pose a small but significant risk to the patient, need be done. For example, where angiography once may have been the procedure of choice in diagnosing intracranial space-occupying lesions, CT scanning and MRI are now available at significantly reduced risk to the patient and physician. This movement away from invasive procedures reduces the physician's risk of liability for bad results from a failure of technique in administering the procedure itself.

Further, newer technology allows a greater yield of useful data from most all procedures, including invasive ones, such that on a risk-versus-benefit analysis, the employment of the procedure is more defensible. Moreover, the quality of the data now available may lessen the risk of misdiagnosis or improper diagnosis. Other benefits to the physician from new technology may be purely economic, in that more and more procedures can be done on an outpatient basis and can be done more expeditiously, allowing processing of a larger number of patients.

The burdens of the new technology, however, are also significant. Identification of disease conditions and pathologic processes, localization of occult disease, and determination of the etiology of the disease have become more efficacious with the use of modern diagnostic radiologic techniques. As a result, the radiologist has become more of a diagnostician. Where once the diagnostic method of choice may have been exploratory surgery, complicated laboratory processes, or the Sherlock Holmes–type deductions drawn therefrom, technology has now to a large extent turned over the investigation to radiologists to employ the relatively inexpensive, low-risk, large-benefit procedures at their fingertips.

The radiologist thus may become the court of last resort for a variety of medical specialists. Because of the latter's concerns about malpractice, such practitioners, on discovering a lump, bump, or other irregularity, may be reluctant to diagnose and treat the condition without the benefits of diagnostic radiology. For example, the general practitioner confronted with a cyst might previously have advised that it merely be followed for changes or that some minor surgical procedure be performed. The prescription now, however, is to send the patient for ultrasonography and see what the radiologist thinks. Given the increased reliance by the clinician and patient on the x-ray results, the potential exposure for malpractice claims necessarily increases.

A second somewhat ironic result of scientific progress concerns the dramatic increase in the ability to treat effectively the once untreatable disease. The medical community as a whole prides itself on doing today what was unthinkable 5 years ago. With an increased ability to treat disease, there is a concomitant pressure on the diagnostician to make the diagnosis so that the new wonders of treatment may be employed. In years past, the failure to diagnose an occult neoplasm did not significantly expose the radiologist to liability, since there was no effective means of treatment anyway. Now, however, there is great potential exposure for failure to make the diagnosis at the earliest possible time so that the patient's life can be saved, or at least significantly lengthened.

The practice of outpatient diagnostic radiology may also be complicated by the very nature of that practice. The radiologist may have very little clinical data with which to work and may have little or no contact with the patient, the actual diagnostic procedure being carried out primarily by technologists. The patients themselves come to the facility, undergo some procedure strange to them, leave without knowing the results, and may not even know the name of the doctor whose diagnostic ability may mean life or death to them.

If something goes wrong in the patient's workup, resulting in significant difficulties for the patient, whom is the patient inclined to blame—the family physician who is known and trusted, or the corporate diagnostic radiology group? In addition, the patient population has increasingly high expectations with regard to the ability to diagnose and treat almost all medical conditions. Thus, when there is arguably a failure of diagnosis, the inclination to believe that such a failure is the result of malpractice may be very great.

The nature and type of errors that may lead to a malpractice claim are as broad as the practice of diagnostic radiology. It may on occasion be the most routine of procedures that results in the malpractice claim. After spending much time with the more sophisticated high-tech procedures, the radiologist may have less interest or inclination to deal with the routine, run-of-the-mill procedure that he or she has been doing for many years. However, a routine x-ray that is given too quick or too casual a reading may result in either a missed diagnosis or a misdiagnosis. Liability has also been imposed for other seemingly fundamental procedures, such as the proper labeling of x-rays. A relevant case involved a situation in which a CT scan was mislabeled so that the right side of the brain was reversed with the left. Although the patient's clinical picture lateralized his brain tumor to a specific side of the brain, surgery was nonetheless carried out on the other side based on the mislabeled CT scans. No tumor was found on that operation, and the patient was forced to undergo a substantial delay in the diagnosis of his tumor. This case demonstrated the great extent to which physicians rely on the results of diagnostic radiology even when the data from those studies do not match the clinical picture.

Obviously, the best method to deal with malpractice problems is to avoid them in the first place. There are some things that practitioners of diagnostic radiology can do to help avoid malpractice claims and to deal with them once they arise. The primary prophylactic agent against malpractice claims probably is the establishment of a quality, caring doctor-patient relationship in which the patient perceives the physician to be genuinely concerned about his or her welfare. This situation may be very difficult to achieve in the practice of outpatient diagnostic radiology, since there may be little doctor-patient contact. [Editor's note: As an adjunct to those times when physician-patient contact is not feasible, we employ a patient coordinator to facilitate the examination of patients, and we also provide each individual with a brochure that has photographs and brief biographies of the center's radiologists.]

As an adjunct to the doctor-patient relationship, the radiologist needs to establish an understanding with the referral base of physicians and institutions. This understanding should somehow be documented to set forth the expectations between the diagnostic radiologist and the referring source, noting what role each will play. The exact nature of the role will vary greatly, no doubt. However, if the diagnostic radiologist is to be used primarily as a tool for the workup of patients by other physicians, some ground rules need to be set about how that tool will be used. To the extent possible, ultimate diagnostic decisions and therapeutic decisions need to be left in the hands of the physicians who have greater access to the patient and to the clinical data. This may be difficult to do in an era when the wonders of technology are so highly touted.

It is also probably a good idea to provide some disclaimer, when appropriate, that the findings reported need to be correlated with the clinical data available. Radiologists need to protect themselves from the referring physician who cannot see past an x-ray report, the results of which may be inconsistent with or directly contradictory to the clinical picture.

Finally, good record keeping is essential, both to document the technical aspects of the procedure performed, especially where it is invasive, and to document the findings and basis for any diagnosis given. Sloppy documentation may imply sloppy work. Precise documentation not only implies precise execution and evaluation of data, but also helps form the basis on which defenses of claims may rest. It is probably impossible for a diagnostic radiologist to remember what happens in every procedure on every patient. Moreover, it is probably impossible to tell which of those patients will end up as a plaintiff against his or her physicians. Therefore, without accurate, complete documentation, the physician may be hard-pressed years after the fact to demonstrate what actually occurred and the basis for diagnoses made. It is better to document the facts when they happen than to speculate about them under cross-examination.

In conclusion, there is logic to the theory that exposure to malpractice claims should decrease with increasingly sophisticated technology. However, technology surely cannot eliminate such claims. In fact, technology may not even reduce claims against physicians and technicians whose practice of diagnostic radiology overemphasizes the wonders of technology and underemphasizes the subtleties of the practice of medicine. It truly is accurate to say that both patients and physicians are exposed to risks in the practice of outpatient diagnostic radiology.

References

1. California, Book of Approved Jury Instructions, 7th ed., Number 6.00, 1986.
2. California, Book of Approved Jury Instructions, 7th ed., Number 6.00, 1986.
3. California, Book of Approved Jury Instructions, 7th ed., Number 6.01, 1986.
4. California, Book of Approved Jury Instructions, 7th ed., Number 6.11, 1986.
5. California, Book of Approved Jury Instructions, 7th ed., Number 6.11.5; Truman v. Thomas, 27 Cal. 3d 285, 1980.

Outpatient Angiography of the Brain, Head, and Neck

Arthur B. Dublin, M.D.

Angiography of the brain, head, and neck has traditionally been performed in an inpatient setting. Although the major complications of these procedures are infrequent, the side effects may be devastating to the patient. In addition, many of these individuals are elderly and consequently may be in poor general health. Despite these drawbacks, outpatient angiography of the brain and adjacent structures can be accomplished safely, with low morbidity and essentially no mortality. Newer catheter materials, improved training at the resident level, less toxic contrast agents, and digital subtraction angiography (DSA) have combined to produce an environment that makes outpatient angiography a safe, reasonably comfortable experience, with reduced cost to the patient and to the health care system as a whole.[1-27] This discussion will outline the appropriate indications and the latest trends for outpatient examinations.

THE EQUIPMENT

The pros and cons of DSA versus conventional film angiography have been discussed at length in the literature.[2-6, 12-14, 28-35] Despite all the rhetoric, the basic question that must be asked is "Does DSA produce images of sufficient quality to answer the majority of clinical questions without increasing patient morbidity or mortality?" The resounding response to this question from our own experience is yes! The literature

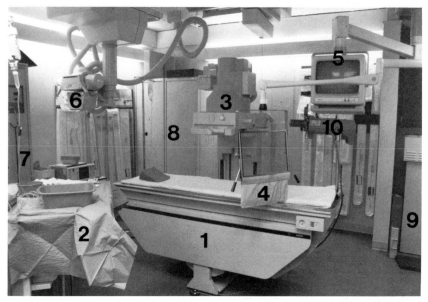

Figure 3–1. Angiographic DSA unit. The various basic components of a DSA angiographic suite are displayed. **1:** Tilt table. **2:** Preparation/procedure tray. **3:** 14-inch image intensifier with 100-mm spot film device. **4:** Face shield. **5:** TV monitor. **6:** Standard overhead x-ray tube. **7:** Med Rad injector control cabinet.* **8:** Power/table power cabinets. **9:** Transformer. **10:** Table-mounted Med Rad power injector.

---

*Med Rad, Inc., 566 Alpha Drive, Pittsburgh, PA 15238

provides additional convincing evidence that this conclusion is justified. This controversy will be discussed in greater detail in this chapter.

The outpatient angiography suite should ideally consist of a biplane fluoroscopic unit with DSA and cut-film backup. However, the cost of such a unit is impractical and prohibitive. In addition, most centers (such as our facility) perform other studies besides angiography, and thus the angiography suite must often do double duty. We use a Philips Diagnost-73* with a plus/minus 90-degree tilt table and a 14/10/6-inch (35.6/25.4/13.2-cm) intensifier supplemented by a 100-mm spot device for use in general fluoroscopy (Fig. 3–1). Although our room is small (14.5 × 16.5 feet), adequate space is available for frequently used supplies, preparation materials, and the variety of catheters and embolic materials employed in both cerebral and general angiographic studies. Patient comfort is enhanced by indirect lighting (direct overhead lighting can be irritating to the patient and may reflect unwanted glare at the angiographer from wet surfaces on the sterile drapes).

---

*Philips Medical Systems, Shelton, Connecticut

Patient position is easily controlled by caudal-cephalad and lateral table motion, allowing a great variety of vascular studies (literally from the head to the toe) to be performed. Most standard and complicated cerebral projections can be obtained by such table movement and by simple head movements (including submentovertex, oblique, and lateral views) (Figs. 3–2 and 3–3). The tilt table is also useful for general fluoroscopy, certain hormonal sampling procedures, and venography (including varicocele embolotherapy) and as an aid in treating vasovagal reactions. The ventilation system should be adjusted so that the angiography room has a cooler-than-normal temperature for the comfort of both the patient and the angiographer. A foot switch interlocked into the room lighting system is helpful for quick conversions from full to subdued lighting.

A table-mounted injector is useful in such small rooms, although such a system may limit the flexibility for extremely angiographic procedures in unusually large patients. However, this injector system is ideal for all head and neck procedures. DSA techniques have eliminated the need for large-volume injections, since 25 ml of 50% diluted contrast agent are almost always satisfactory for aortic arch injections.

The 100-mm spot device can also be used to produce cerebral film subtraction angiography, should the DSA unit malfunction. Both the Philips DVI2 system and 100-mm spot device produce standard exposure rates (both DSA and 100 mm) of up to six frames or exposures per second. However, if desired, a cardiac package can increase this rate to 30 frames per second. The radiation exposure measured at the face of the fluoroscope is 100 to 125 microrems per frame per 100-mm work and 150 to 175 microrems for digital examinations.

CONVENTIONAL PLAIN FILM ANGIOGRAPHY VERSUS INTRAARTERIAL DIGITAL SUBTRACTION ANGIOGRAPHY

Plain film (PF) angiography has been the mainstay of cerebral radiographic investigations for many years. Improvements in film changer technology have produced a reliable filming system with a high spatial resolution (5 to 6 line pairs/mm).[11, 30] Despite the fact that PF angiography may be performed advantageously in an outpatient setting, intraarterial DSA (IADSA) offers several benefits that are particularly promising for outpatient techniques.[2, 6, 12–15, 28–36]

It has been my experience and that of other investigators that IADSA, although somewhat inferior to PF filming in regard to spatial resolution (IADSA, 2 to 3 line pairs/mm with a 6-inch field and a 512×512 matrix), is superior in so many other aspects as to be the method of choice for

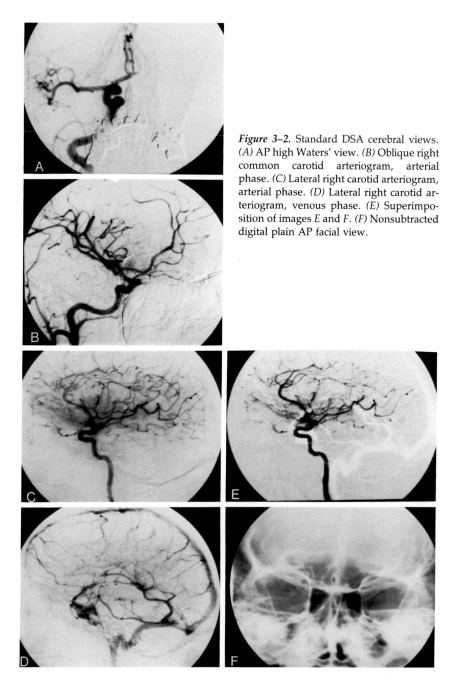

Figure 3–2. Standard DSA cerebral views. *(A)* AP high Waters' view. *(B)* Oblique right common carotid arteriogram, arterial phase. *(C)* Lateral right carotid arteriogram, arterial phase. *(D)* Lateral right carotid arteriogram, venous phase. *(E)* Superimposition of images *E* and *F*. *(F)* Nonsubtracted digital plain AP facial view.

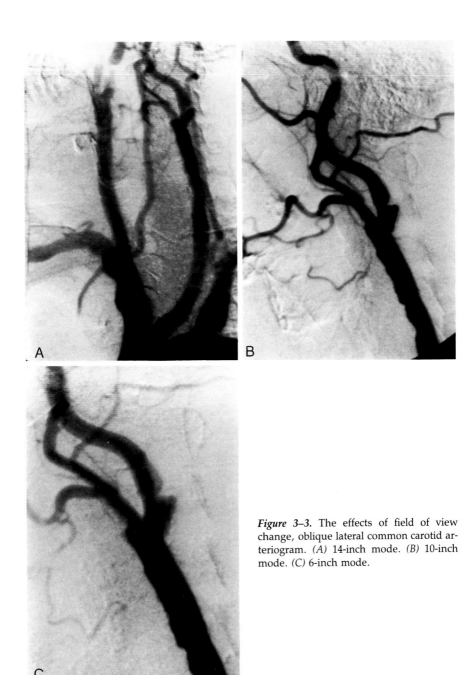

Figure 3–3. The effects of field of view change, oblique lateral common carotid arteriogram. *(A)* 14-inch mode. *(B)* 10-inch mode. *(C)* 6-inch mode.

Table 3–1
COMPARISON OF PLAIN FILM TECHNIQUES
VERSUS IADSA

	Plain Film	IADSA
Spatial resolution	Better	Worse
Contrast resolution	Worse	Better
Cost per exam	Worse	Better
Cost of equipment	Worse	Better
Patient discomfort from standard contrast agents	Worse	Better
Filming rate	Worse	Better
Availability of subtraction films	Worse	Better
Field coverage	Same for head work	

cerebral, head, and neck evaluations.[12, 30, 34] Table 3–1 compares the advantages of PF angiography and IADSA. IADSA is superior in providing the rapid acquisition of subtracted images for review. The latter is especially important during embolic procedures to monitor the progress of successful embolic flow changes.[37] Faster frame rates are available with IADSA (up to 30 frames/second) as compared with PF angiography. The field of view may be changed more rapidly with IADSA than with PF angiography (Fig. 3–3). The Philips unit in our facility can superimpose a static contrast image on real-time fluoroscopy, producing a "road map" of anatomy for reference during embolic work. This map can also serve as an aid in the successful catheterization of difficult anatomic variations. Because of the diminished volumes and concentrations of contrast agents necessary to produce diagnostic images with IADSA, patient motion is reduced, and thus the "effective" spatial resolution of IADSA may actually be superior to PF angiography in certain cases.

IADSA is superior in contrast resolution (0.2% contrast resolution or 2 to 3% iodine concentration) compared with PF angiography (2% contrast resolution, or 40 to 50% iodine concentration).[38] Therefore, IADSA enables better detection of peripheral or slower flowing portions of arteriovenous malformations and provides a superior tumor stain. Other slow-flow situations, such as in high-grade carotid stenosis, may be enhanced with IADSA.[39] According to Mani and colleagues, the size of the catheter, the patient's age, and the length of the examination all increase the risk of stroke during cerebral angiography.[40-42] IADSA examination is quick, allows the use of smaller catheters and decreased amounts of contrast agents, and thus theoretically decreases the risk of stroke complications.

The cost savings may be considerable with IADSA. We use a six-on-one filming format on a 14 × 17-inch single-emulsion film. In our experience, four such 14 × 17-inch films are adequate to image the pertinent information of a typical bilateral carotid artery and aortic arch study, for

Table 3–2
COMPARISON OF COSTS OF SELECTED CONTRAST AGENTS
(Based on an Average of 100 ml per Exam)

	g/ml	ml	$/Bottle	$/g
Iodine				
Conray 300*	141	300	7.87	0.19
Isovue†	300	50	45.99	3.06
Omnipaque‡	300	50	45.90	3.06
Hexabrix*	320	50	50.60	3.16

Note: Nonionic materials can be diluted 50% to obtain comparable iodine concentrations and adequate volume for a standard cerebrovascular examination.

*Mallinckrodt, Inc., St. Louis, Missouri
†Squibb Diagnostics, New Brunswick, New Jersey
‡Winthrop-Breon Labs, New York, New York

a total film cost of $7.92.* A typical PF examination of the same anatomy uses 56 14 × 14-inch double-sided emulsion films, for a total cost of $72.24.† Thus, the savings in film costs for every 100 such patients is $6,432. Weinstein and colleagues suggest a greater savings, $140, for every complete cervicocerebral study if digital techniques are used in place of PF angiography.[43] For more complicated cases, the savings increase proportionately. Many other centers have cited similar dramatic decreases in conventional film use (80% in one instance over a period of 6 months) since the introduction of IADSA.[30] The potential cost savings attributable to the use of dilute ionic contrast agents are outlined in Table 3–2.

The limitations of IADSA are few.[1] The field of view of most image intensifiers is smaller than that provided by PF angiography, a factor to be considered in the evaluation of abdominal and extremity vascular structures. However, larger-sized screens (14 inches or greater) are now available to cover all body parts more adequately. For head and neck work, our 6- and 10-inch modes are used most frequently, and such formats are available with most units in operation. Increased resolution is possible with newer 1024 × 1024 matrix units, but the 512 × 512 format is more than satisfactory for the vast majority of IADSA examinations. Motion artifacts produced by pharyngeal motion (accentuated by calcified plaques) are only infrequently a serious problem. Electrocardiogram (ECG)-synchronized exposure control can improve image quality in these latter situations.[44] PF angiography is indicated for the very uncooperative individual who is not a candidate for DSA.

---

*Cronex MRF 33, E.I. du Pont de Nemours & Co., Inc., Wilmington, Delaware
†Cronex 7, E.I. du Pont de Nemours & Co., Inc., Wilmington, Delaware

INTRAVENOUS VERSUS INTRAARTERIAL DIGITAL SUBTRACTION ANGIOGRAPHY

IVDSA was initially thought to be a major breakthrough in angiographic technique.[2, 6, 29-31] Unfortunately, IVDSA has not, as a whole, lived up to this promise.[4-6, 12-15, 33-36] Even the major centers that pioneered IVDSA techniques now admit that IADSA has become the preferred mode of investigation of head, neck, and cerebrovascular disease.[30] Table 3–3 summarizes the pros and cons of intraarterial versus intravenous examinations.

IVDSA does have several advantages, including the lack of intraarterial embolic complications, a reduced level of technical skill required for the performance of the study, less patient-interaction time necessary for the radiologist, and decreased recovery time.[30-31] However, IVDSA has several disadvantages as well.[2, 4, 12, 30, 33, 35-36] Most individuals undergoing an assessment of the carotid and vertebral arterial supply often have multisystem atheromatous disease, affecting the heart. Thus, this class of patients often has a poor cardiac output and therefore a reduced capability to maintain a superior bolus effect of the contrast agent as it passes from the venous to the arterial side of the circulation, with resultant image degradation.[6, 45] In addition, these patients are often elderly and are therefore less likely to be able to remain still during the circulation of contrast agent into the arterial vasculature, a crucial point in obtaining optimal subtraction images.[12]

Multiple projections may be necessary because of anatomic variations, which may produce overlap of the carotid bifurcations (Fig. 3–4).[46] Therefore, since IVDSA studies are usually confined to three to five injections per study because of contrast limits, the evaluation of the carotid circulation may be incomplete and suboptimal.[30] In addition, IVDSA injections are not without side effects and produce a higher rate of allergic reaction and hyperemesis (which may degrade the images) than do IADSA studies.[47] In addition, IVDSA has been reported as causing angina, congestive

Table 3–3
COMPARISON OF IVDSA VERSUS IADSA

	IVDSA	IADSA
Contrast resolution	Worse	Better
Spatial resolution	Worse	Better
Embolic risk to brain	None	Worse
Cost	Equivalent	
Patient recovery	Better	Worse
Decreased contrast loads with lessened cardiac effects	Worse	Better
Patient interaction required by physician	Less	More

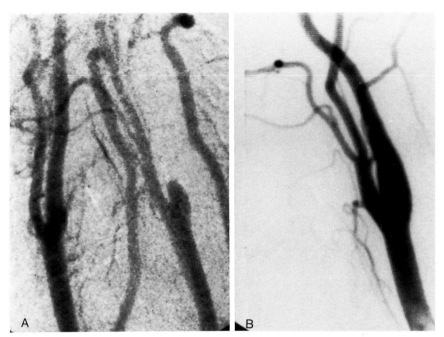

Figure 3–4. IVDSA versus IADSA. Superimposition of vessels with IVDSA *(A)* and the decreased contrast-to-noise ratio may produce suboptimal studies when compared with a selected carotid injection with IADSA *(B)*.

heart failure, arrhythmias, and myocardial ischemia.[48–49] Chest pain without ischemia or infarction and hypotension from extravasation of contrast agents from the superior vena cava (SVC) and right atrium have also been described.[30, 50] Transient ischemic attacks (TIAs) also have been reported following IVDSA, presumably on the basis of cerebral hypoxia or contrast toxicity.[30, 51] Finally, the simple peripheral vein injection has evolved into a right atrial injection technique, all in an attempt to increase the quality of the images.[30, 50]

IADSA has multiple advantages as compared with IVDSA, including superior contrast resolution; decreased contrast load; decreased cerebral, cardiac, and renal toxicity; and reduced motion artifacts caused by swallowing, nausea, and vomiting.[12, 30, 33–36] In addition, there is less vascular overlap with IADSA as compared with IVDSA. IADSA does require more physician interaction, but some radiologists consider the latter a bonus rather than a disadvantage in that closer patient-physician relationships are established, possibly leading to better communication, better examinations, and better postprocedure follow-up compliance.

IADSA is extremely useful for embolic procedures. Subtracted images can be obtained rapidly, and the superb contrast resolution allows excellent visualization of superselected facial vessels (Fig. 3–5). Stereoscopic

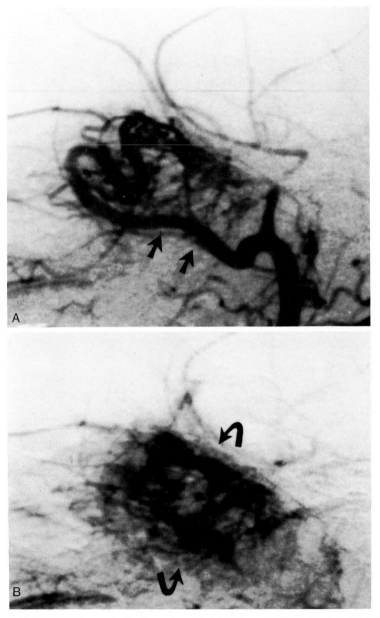

Figure 3–5. Preoperative embolization of nasal juvenile angiofibroma. Arterial *(A)* and capillary *(B)* phases, lateral view of the external carotid artery demonstrate an enlarged internal maxillary artery (IMA) (arrows), and a tumor blush (curved arrows), typical of an angiofibroma.

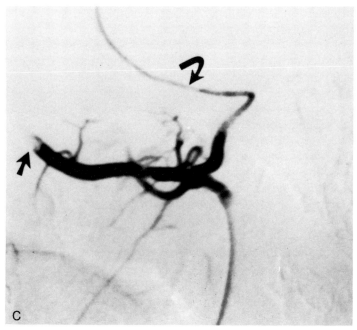

Figure 3–5 *Continued (C)* Post embolization. A subselective injection into the IMA shows very little tumor stain, occlusion of the distal IMA (arrow), and preservation of the middle meningeal artery (curved arrow).

and tomographic IADSA are experimental techniques that may have future practical applications for routine cerebrovascular procedures.[52–54]

TECHNIQUE OF THE BASIC CEREBROVASCULAR EXAMINATION

Intravenous Digital Subtraction Angiography

As stated above, IVDSA is inferior in many respects to IADSA. However, IVDSA may be useful in certain limited circumstances (e.g., poor arterial access routes) and thus will be briefly discussed. IVDSA is ideally performed using a high-flow 4 or 5 French pigtail catheter, most commonly placed via an antecubital vein into the right atrium. Hicks and colleagues demonstrated the advantages of a centrally placed bolus into the right atrium, versus a more peripheral injection with the catheter tip in an antecubital vein position.[6] The former improved the peak concentration of contrast (63%, peripheral vein; 85%, superior vena cava; right atrium, 100%).[3, 38, 45] If spasm is encountered, an infusion of dextrose or saline solution for a few minutes may alleviate this problem. A full-strength, high-concentration material such as Renografin-76* (30 to 50 ml total at 35 ml/second), or newer nonionic materials should be used.[30] However, the cost factor of nonionic agents may be prohibitive (Table 3–2). Increasing the rate of delivery of contrast beyond 35 ml/second has little effect on the image contrast quality, especially if the cardiac output is poor. In addition, osmolarity and viscosity have no effect on the final iodine concentration.[45] The total volume injected during a procedure should be limited to 200 ml or less, which is especially important if the exacerbation of previously unknown renal disease is to be avoided.[30]

Seeger and Carmody suggest a schema for the selection of IVDSA technique.[30] If an asymptomatic carotid bruit is present, Doppler ultrasonography should be performed first. If the Doppler results are normal, then no further imaging techniques should be used. If the Doppler examination is positive, IVDSA should be undertaken. If a definite TIA in a single or multiple anatomic territory is present, then IADSA is indicated. The latter is particularly true for vertebrobasilar disease, since IVDSA is suboptimal for this anatomic region. However, the role and accuracy of Doppler ultrasonography in the evaluation of carotid disease are controversial.[55–61] In our experience, Doppler is often erroneous, even in the best of hands. The majority of patients with asymptomatic carotid bruits do not develop symptoms. Therefore, carotid Doppler examination certainly is not indicated if a nonoperative, conservative management program is recommended for asymptomatic carotid lesions.[62–64] If the patient is symptomatic, then angiography will eventually be performed, and thus the role of ultrasonography in this latter group is also questionable.

Careful coaching of the patient regarding breath holding, swallowing, and head motion all can help to improve the IVDSA examination. Topical pharyngeal xylocaine may be beneficial to combat the heat sensation and swallowing reflex produced by ionic materials, although the newer nonionic contrast agents have eliminated much of the perception of heat and pain.[16–27, 30] An average delay of 4 seconds from the start of the injection to the beginning of the filming sequence is recommended. However, poor cardiac function may produce longer delays of up to 10 seconds or more. An exposure rate of two per second is quite sufficient, but for individuals with decreased cardiac output, one exposure per second may be satisfactory.

Wagner and associates and Faerber and colleagues described their experiences using IVDSA in children.[65–66] Chloral hydrate (50 to 100 mg/kg) or a cocktail of meperidine (Demerol) (2 mg/kg), promethazine (Phenergan) (0.5 mg/kg), and chlorpromazine (Thorazine) (2 mg/kg) were used for sedation. Although this approach was successful in many cases,

*Squibb Diagnostic Inc., New Brunswick, New Jersey

intravenous ketamine had to be used as a supplement, and in general, young children should be treated as inpatients. There are exceptions, and on occasion we have performed examinations on mature children with little or no preexamination sedation.

Intraarterial Digital Subtraction Angiography

IADSA is our preferred method of investigating head and neck pathology. The ideal site for the introduction of the catheter is controversial. Hicks and colleagues suggest that there is no difference in the rate of central nervous system (CNS) complications between the transbrachial and the transfemoral route.[6] Furthermore, Hicks states that there are insufficient data to evaluate local complications of arterial thrombosis secondary to arterial spasm using the transbrachial approach. He further suggests that data showing a higher complication rate with the transbrachial route are based on a brachial artery cutdown technique and the use of large 7 or 8 French catheters. The transbrachial approach has the advantage of a shorter recovery period, and it is especially useful for carotid and vertebral catheterizations that are technically impossible from the femoral approach.

Nevertheless, we (as well as many other authors) prefer the transfemoral technique for routine head and neck cases.[30, 33] The latter approach provides easier access for the selection of all cerebral vessels, avoids the blind passage of a catheter through diseased subclavian and innominate arteries, and may have a lessened complication rate overall as compared with the transbrachial route.[6, 30] Seeger and Carmody suggest a 4 French pigtail catheter for the arch injection, using 20 to 24 ml total at 12 ml/second of 60% Conray.* For selective carotid or vertebral injections, they recommend a 4.5 or 5 French cerebral catheter using 6 to 7 ml of 43% Conray at 4 to 5 ml/second per injection.[30] In our experience, a 5 French catheter (Fig. 3–6) is sufficient for both arch and selective studies. A 4 French catheter is less effective in older individuals because of poorer catheter torque control. We employ 25 ml of 30% Conray at 12 ml/second for the aortic arch view and 4 to 5 ml total of the same agent at 3 to 4 ml/second for selective common carotid arterial injections. A double-ended wire (straight and 5 mm J)* or a movable-core 0.035-inch J curve or straight wire is very useful. A 5 French straight catheter† may be formed into unusual curves with steam and is helpful in catheterizing difficult arterial curves. A 5 French Berenstein-type curve† is extremely useful for embolic work or for selecting the vertebral artery. It is extremely unusual to have to resort to a Simmons-type J catheter† or a larger 6.5 or 7 French

*Argon Medical Corp., Athens, Texas
†Cook Inc., Bloomington, Indiana

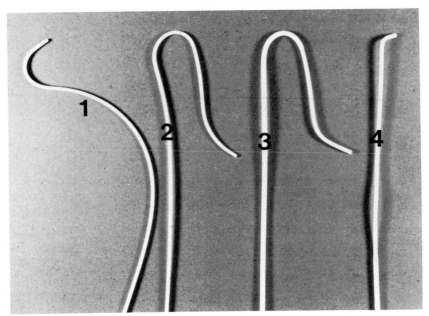

Figure 3–6. Recommended catheter types for cerebral and head and neck studies. **1**: JB-2 5 French. **2**: Simmons 5 French. **3**: Simmons 5/7 French. **4**: Berenstein 5/7—"hockey stick."

catheter,* except in rare cases of severe vessel tortuosity, femoral bleeding about a smaller-sized catheter, or poor torque control of the catheter material due to vessel tortuosity. Figure 3–7 shows our customary preparation tray for a standard cervicocerebral angiogram.

Newer agents such as Hexabrix,* Omnipaque,† and Isovue‡ all are supposedly less toxic and more comfortable than standard ionic agents such as Conray.[16–27] However, IADSA allows the use of decreased volumes and concentrations of ionic agents. Therefore, in our experience, the acceptability of ionic materials is greatly increased, with little if any discomfort experienced by the patient. In addition, the toxic load of ionic agents is greatly reduced with IADSA. The comparisons of nonionic with ionic contrast materials in the literature are based on full strengths of ionic material. It is unclear whether the advantages of nonionic agents over ionic compounds such as Conray exist at more dilute concentrations and decreased total volumes. Table 3–2 lists the relative costs of nonionic compounds and 30% Conray.

*Mallinckrodt, Inc., St. Louis, Missouri
†Winthrop-Breon, New York, New York
‡Squibb Diagnostic, Inc., New Brunswick, New Jersey

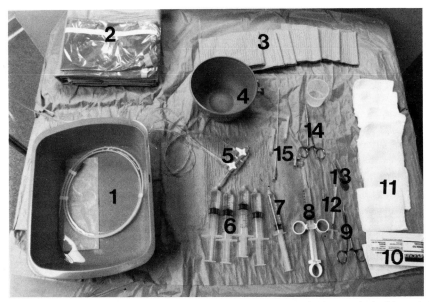

Figure 3–7. Standard angiographic procedure tray. **1:** Heparinized saline with double-ended wire, telfa strip pad. **2:** Sterile patient drape. **3:** Paper towels. **4:** Flush discard bowl. **5:** Double stopcock system for heparinized saline flush and contrast agent. **6:** Flush syringes. **7:** Contrast. **8:** Local anesthesia. **9:** Curved Kelly clamp. **10:** Image-intensifier drape. **11:** Gauze. **12:** Seldinger needle. **13:** Number 11 blade. **14:** Straight Kelly clamp. **15:** One-way stopcock, 5 French dilator, hypodermic needles.

Preparation for the Standard Head and Neck Exam

The patient is instructed to continue any usual medications and to drink ample fluids the night and morning before the study. Diabetics should drink juices for sugar intake and use insulin per routine. Dextrose should not be used for diabetics during the procedure, and ½ normal saline is substituted instead. A responsible adult should be readily available for transportation to home following the recovery process. No premedications are given, except for the unusually anxious individual. An intravenous line is started in all patients in the left (side away from the angiographer) arm, a blood pressure cuff is placed on the right arm, and ECG monitoring leads are placed in such a manner so as not to obscure aortic or neck vascular detail. If the patient is not already taking aspirin or similar antiplatelet agents, two 5-grain aspirins are administered at least 1 hour before the start of the procedure.[5, 67]

A Seldinger double-wall femoral arterial puncture technique is used, and a JB2 5 French catheter is primarily used for aortic and selective examinations. An exposure rate of two frames per second is used for both the standard arch and selective carotid views, but the rate can be increased to six frames per second on our unit for the examination of fistulas, arteriovenous malformations (AVMs), and vascular tumors. A face shield is desired for hand injections, when the latter are necessary (e.g., embolic procedures or tenuous selective catheterizations). A left anterior oblique projection is used for the aortic arch (10- or 14-inch mode). Both oblique views are occasionally used, especially if selective catheterization of the carotid or vertebral vessels is not contemplated or feasible. A 10-inch mode is usually sufficient for frontal and lateral projections (which simultaneously show the intracranial and extracranial vascular structures). The 6-inch mode is used as needed for more detailed intra- or extracranial studies.

The Recovery Process

In our facility, a three-bed recovery suite is sufficient to serve the entire department, including hospital transfers who are waiting for noninvasive examinations, and for postprocedure recovery for all types of invasive procedures. Following a venous or arterial examination, the patient is promptly removed to the recovery area, and using syringe aspiration or occasionally a guide wire, the catheter is withdrawn. Manual pressure is applied for 10 minutes. We prefer not to rely on a sandbag for femoral compression, since this technique is uncomfortable for the patient and may produce undesired motion. In addition, the sandbag may give the angiographer a false sense of security and is no guarantee against a significant hematoma. For larger facilities, a nurse may be useful to perform the observation procedure. We monitor the patient using a nonnurse patient coordinator, supplemented by periodic visits by the angiographer. After the observation period (1 to 2 hours for transbrachial, 3 hours for a transfemoral approach), the patient is taken by wheelchair to the mode of transportation home, with instructions for bed rest for the remainder of the day but with resumption of usual activities (aside from vigorous athletics) the following day. A contact telephone number is also given to the patient, along with specific warnings regarding delayed complications.

Complications

Most complications from intraarterial procedures (contrast reaction, neurologic deficit, leg ischemia, and excessive bleeding) occur immediately or within 1 to 2 hours after the examination.[68] Delayed complications are extremely unlikely to occur if the peripheral pulses are unchanged from their preexamination status.[69] Pseudoaneurysm formation is generally not appreciated until days or weeks after the study. Therefore, routine overnight inpatient observation of patients is not likely to affect the rate or outcome of complications. Hospitalization should be reserved for patients with significant postangiography complications and for patients with uncontrolled hypertension, bleeding disorders, or renal disease. Uncooperative individuals incapable of providing appropriate follow-up by themselves or by a relative also are candidates for hospitalization.[3]

Mani and colleagues reviewed 5,000 intraarterial cerebral angiograms performed in a hospital setting.[40–42] The main factors increasing the risk of significant complication were advanced patient age, extended length of time for the study, and larger catheter size. IADSA has decreased the risk of the latter two factors by allowing smaller catheter sizes for decreased contrast loads and by decreasing the time for a typical examination.

Wolfel and colleagues reported a 0.3% major complication rate in 2,029 outpatient arterial studies (performed in a variety of anatomic regions), one-third of the rate encountered by inpatient examinations at his facility.[7] However, the inpatient population may have been in poorer health than the outpatient group. In addition, Wolfel had no residents performing the outpatient studies (Mani suggested that the university setting with resident trainees had a higher complication rate than the private hospital).[7–9, 11, 40–42]

Saint-Georges and associates reported the results of 100 patients with a variety of general and neurovascular vascular procedures, examined in an outpatient setting.[1] Ninety-four were discharged within 4 hours of the study and were still well 1 week later. One patient was hospitalized with oliguria (released 10 days later, progressing well), whereas five others were kept under observation for transient hypotension, hematoma, abdominal pain, or a combination thereof. They were eventually also released and progressed well. The catheter site (8 French) may have been a contributing factor in producing the complications in three of these cases.

Adams and Roub reported on 143 outpatient angiograms (17% of total angiograms performed).[11] Seventy-nine were accomplished from the femoral approach, with 46 examinations of the aortic arch, carotids, or vertebrals (no complications).[11] Brown and colleagues reported only one minor complication (a small groin hematoma, no treatment necessary) and no major complications in 75 consecutive patients undergoing outpatient cerebral IADSA.[4]

Bank used a 4 French catheter technique and IADSA in 400 outpatients (87% neurovascular).[5] In his first 200 cases (no aspirin by mouth), five transient visual or visual/aphasia complications were observed, along with one permanent aphasia. After the routine administration of two tablets of

Table 3–4
NEUROVASCULAR COMPLICATIONS

		Number of Patients	Number/% of Complications
Bank et al.		348	5/1.4%
Brown et al.		72	1/1.4%
Dublin		200	3/1.5%
	Total	620	9/1.5%

aspirin orally before the study, no neurologic complications were observed in the next 200 patients. Of the total 400 cases, one large, two moderate, and four small hematomas were encountered, none of which required hospitalization.[5]

Finally, our own experience confirms the safety of IADSA outpatient angiography. Two complications (2%) were encountered in our first 100 patients (80% of the total cases), including one case of homonymous hemianopsia (transient, 15 minutes, complete recovery) and one brief episode of vasovagal reaction. A summary of these authors' experience is listed in Table 3–4.

EMBOLIC TECHNIQUES

Most intracranial embolic techniques are best performed in an inpatient setting because of the critical nature of the pathologies that require such techniques (e.g., intracranial AVMs, fistulas). However, there are certain extracranial and pericranial lesions that may be safely embolized in an outpatient setting. These pathologies include primarily chemodectomas, juvenile angiofibromas, facial vascular lesions, and meningiomas. We have also embolized a nasal bleeder, although this was a hospital transfer.

The preparation of the patient is the same as for routine procedures, with the exception that the consent process is more detailed, and pre-medication with intramuscular meperidine (75 to 100 mg) and atropine (0.5 mg) may be given on occasion for the control of pain and vasovagal reactions, respectively.

The external carotid artery is usually the artery to be catheterized for embolotherapy. Because of the multiple branches that may supply any given lesion, a standard cerebral catheter such as the Cook JB2 may not be satisfactory for this technique. We have found that a "hockey-stick" type distal tip, either preformed* or steam formed at the time of the study, can be very helpful in superselective examinations.

The choice of embolic material depends on the type of pathology to be treated. For instance, occluding spring emboli* (Fig. 3–8) are useful for

---

*Cook, Inc., Bloomington, Indiana

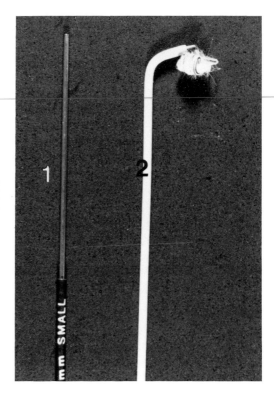

Figure 3–8. Embolization coil. **1:** The coil in introducer sheath. **2:** The coil released by a guide wire via a delivery catheter.

larger-vessel occlusion (e.g., a lacerated internal maxillary artery) or as a final treatment in the embolization of a juvenile angiofibroma.[70] One disadvantage is the inability to "float" coils into position. The catheter must be in exact proximity to the final occluding level.

Particulate materials, introduced either as commercially prepared powders (polyvinyl alcohol foam [PVAF]* or Gelfoam†) (Fig. 3–9) or cut into desired fragments at the time of the study, are preferred for the embolotherapy of hypervascular tumors.[71–72] PVAF is a permanent embolic substance that has a tendency to clump in the catheter or syringe. Gelfoam is an absorbable product and therefore may not be suitable for long-term palliation of lesions. Gelfoam has a lower coefficient of friction than PVAF; therefore, a combination of these two materials may be the best compromise. Certainly, Gelfoam is sufficient as a preoperative embolic tool if the surgery is not delayed longer than 1 week from the embolization.

Whatever material is used, the embolotherapy of facial and accessible intracranial tumors should consist of two major components: (1) occlusion of the tumor bed by fine particles (50 to 300 microns) and (2) embolization

*Unipoint Labs, High Point, North Carolina
†Upjohn Co., Kalamazoo, Michigan

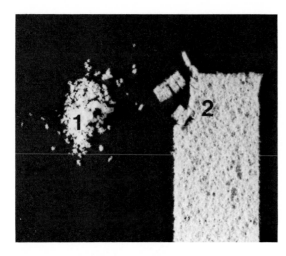

Figure 3–9. Embolic materials. **1:** Polyvinyl alcohol powder. **2:** Gelfoam sponge with partially formed emboli.

of major feeders with larger pledgets of PVAF or Gelfoam sponge. If 2 precedes 1, deeper collaterals may arise and can actually worsen the surgical approach.[73] A waiting period of 3 to 5 days prior to the surgical removal of hypervascular tumors may promote tumor shrinkage.[71] The emboli are introduced with half-strength 30% Conray, which is easily seen with IADSA. If more concentrated solutions are needed, the newer nonionic materials may be used instead of Conray to minimize the pain of the superselective injection.[16–27] However, in our experience, pain has not been a problem with the use of Conray. An IADSA is mandatory following every one to two emboli injections, to detect the earliest filling of contrast into intracranial vessels, either by reflux or by collateral supply.[71]

Dural AVMs are commonly supplied by the middle meningeal artery or by dural branches from the ascending pharyngeal or occipital arteries. Glomus tumors have variable supplies, usually primarily from the ascending pharyngeal artery. Nasopharyngeal angiofibromas typically are supplied by the internal maxillary artery but may have muscular branches from the vertebral artery, especially in the postoperative recurrence (Fig. 3–5).

Complications are rare but may include inadvertent introduction of emboli into intracerebral territories, paresis of a variety of cranial nerves (e.g., the seventh following occipital arterial occlusion), and skin necrosis.[71, 75] To avoid such seventh-nerve paralysis, the catheter tip should be positioned beyond the level of the mastoid process.

CONCLUSION

Outpatient angiography of the brain, head, and neck is a safe and appropriate technique for a great majority of patients with cerebrovascular disease and head and neck tumors. IADSA plays a prominent role in the performance of these studies and allows embolization therapy to be accomplished more easily in a selected number of patients.

References

1. Saint-Georges G, Aube M: Safety of outpatient angiography: A prospective study. AJR 144:235–236, 1985.
2. Becker GJ, Hicks ME, Holden RW: Patient selection, catheters, and contrast agents in intravenous and intra-arterial DSA. Part 2. Appl Radiol Jan/Feb, 69–73, 1986.
3. Jahnke RW, Spencer RS: Why arteriography is going the outpatient route. Diag Imag Mar, 66–69, 1985.
4. Brown PA, Osborn AG, Harnsberger HR, et al: Outpatient intra-arterial digital angiography. West Neuroradiol Soc Ann Meet (Santa Barbara), 1984.
5. Bank WO: Outpatient Angiography. West Neuroradiol Soc Ann Meet (Santa Barbara), 1984.
6. Hicks ME, Becker GJ, Holden R: Better catheters, contrast contribute to DSA's growth. Diagn Imag Jan, 74–80, 1985.
7. Wolfel DA, Lovett BP, Ortenburger AL, et al: Outpatient arteriography: Its safety and cost effectiveness. Radiology 153:363–364, 1985.
8. Giustra PE, Killoran PJ: Outpatient arteriography at a small community hospital. Radiology 116:581–583, 1975.
9. Giustra PE, Killoran PJ: Outpatient arteriography. J Maine Med Assoc 67:124–125, 1976.
10. Fritz AL, et al: Femoral intra-arterial digital angiography: An outpatient procedure. AJR 141:593–596, 1983.
11. Adams PS Jr, Roub LW: Outpatient angiography and interventional radiology: Safety and cost benefits. Radiology 151:81–82, 1984.
12. Foley WD, Milde MW: Intra-arterial digital subtraction angiography. Radiol Clin North Am 23:293–319, 1985.
13. Kelly W, Brant-Zawadski M, Pitts LH: Arterial injection-digital subtraction angiography. J Neurosurg 58:851–856, 1983.
14. Earnest F IV, Houser OW, Forbes GS, et al: The accuracy and limitations of intravenous digital subtraction angiography in the evaluation of atherosclerotic cerebrovascular disease: Angiographic and surgical correlations. Mayo Clin Proc 58:735–746, 1983.
15. Bunker SR, Cutaia FI, Fritz AL, et al: Femoral intra-arterial digital angiography: An outpatient procedure. AJR 141:593–596, 1983.
16. Sackett JF, Bergsjordet B, Seeger JF, et al: Digital subtraction angiography: Comparison of meglumine-Na diatrizoate with iohexol. Acta Radiol (Suppl) 366:81–84, 1983.
17. Cacayorin ED, Bernstein AD, Fruehan CT, et al: Intravenous digital subtraction angiography with iohexol. AJNR 4:329–332, 1983.
18. Amundsen P, Dugstad G, Presthus J, et al: Randomized double-blind cross-over study of iohexol and amnipaque in cerebral angiography. AJNR 4:342–343, 1983.
19. Bryan RN, Miller SL, Roehm JOF Jr, et al: Neuroangiography with iohexol. AJNR 4:344–346, 1983.
20. Hindmarsh T, Bergstrand G, Ericson K, et al: Comparative double-blind investigation of meglumine metrizoate, metrizamide, and iohexol in carotid angiography. AJNR 4:347–349, 1983.
21. Cronqvist S: Iohexol in cerebral angiography; survey and present state. Acta Radiol (Suppl) 366:135–139, 1983.
22. Schonfeld SM, Pinto RS, Schonfeld AR, et al: Iopamidol and Conray 60: Comparison in superselective angiography. Radiology 152:809–811, 1984.

23. Drayer BP, Velaj R, Bird R, et al: Comparative safety of intracranial iopamidol, iothalamate meglumine and diatrizoate meglumine for cerebral angiography. Invest Radiol (Suppl) 19:212–218, 1984.
24. Pelz D, Fox AJ, Vinuela F: Clinical trial of ionexol versus Conray 60 for cerebral angiography. AJNR 5:565–568, 1984.
25. Matozzi F, Turski PA, Gentry LR, et al: Cerebral angiography. Clinical comparison of iopamidol and Conray-60. Invest Radiol (Suppl) 19:219–221, 1984.
26. Norman D, Brant-Zawadzki M, Sobel D: Tolerability and efficacy of Hexabrix in cerebral angiography. Invest Radiol (Suppl) 19:306–307, 1984.
27. Robertson WD, Nugent RA, Russell DB, et al: Clinical experience with hexabrix in cerebral angiography. Invest Radiol (Suppl) 19:308–311, 1984.
28. Muroff LR, Mazer MJ, Eikman EA, et al: Pros and cons of digital radiography vs. plain film debated. Radiol Today 2:3,8, 1985.
29. Hesselink JR: Indications for DSA in neuroradiology. Appl Radiol Jul/Aug, 38–44, 1984.
30. Seeger JF, Carmody RF: Digital subtraction angiography of the arteries of the head and neck. Radiol Clin North Am 23:193–210, 1985.
31. Johnson CM, Sheedy PF, Earnest F IV, et al: Digital subtraction angiography. Surg Clin North Am 64:151–171, 1984.
32. Gardeur D, Seurott M, Fonda C, et al: Digital intravenous subtraction angiography of intracranial arteriovenous malformations. Neuroradiology 25:307–313, 1984.
33. Osborn AG, Edwards MK: Guidelines for using IADSA as a screening procedure cited. Radiol Today 2:7,14, 1985.
34. McCreary JA, Schelhas KP, Brant-Zawadzki M, et al: Outpatient DSA in cerebrovascular disease using transbrachial arch injections. AJR 145:941–947, 1985.
35. Davis PC, Hoffman JC: Work in progress. Intra-arterial digital subtraction angiography: Evaluation in 150 patients. Radiology 149:9–15, 1983.
36. Turski PA, Zwiebel WV, Strother CM, et al: Limitations of intravenous digital subtraction angiography. AJNR 4:271–273, 1983.
37. Kerber CW: Flow-controlled therapeutic embolization: A physiologic and safe technique. AJNR 1:77–81, 1980.
38. Saddekni S, Sos TA, Srur M, et al: Contrast administration and techniques of digital subtraction angiography performance. Radiol Clin North Am 23:275–291, 1985.
39. Gabrielson TO, Seeger JF, Knake JE, et al: The nearly occluded internal carotid artery: A diagnostic trap. Radiology 138:611–618, 1981.
40. Mani RL, Eisenberg RL, McDonald EJ Jr, et al: Complications of catheter cerebral arteriography: Analysis of 5,000 procedures. I. Criteria and incidence. AJR 131:861–865, 1978.
41. Mani RL, Eisenberg RL: Complications of catheter cerebral arteriography: Analysis of 5,000 procedures. II. Relation of complication rates to clinical and arteriographic diagnosis. AJR 113:867–869, 1978.
42. Mani RL, Eisenberg RL: Complications of catheter cerebral arteriography: Analysis of 5,000 procedures. III. Assessment of arteries injected, contrast medium used, duration of procedure, and age of patient. AJR 131:871–874, 1978.
43. Weinstein MA, Pavlicek WA, Modic MI, et al: Intra-arterial digital subtraction angiography of head and neck. Radiology 147:717–724, 1983.
44. Kelly WM, Gould R, Norman D, et al: ECG-synchronized DSA exposure control: Improved cervicothoracic image quality. AJNR 5:429–432, 1984.
45. Burbank FH: Determinants of contrast enhancement for intravenous digital subtraction angiography. Invest Radiol 18:308–316, 1983.
46. Kaseff LG: Positional variations of the common carotid artery bifurcation: Implications for digital subtraction angiography. Radiology 145:377–378, 1982.

47. Sheldon JJ, Janowitz W, Leborque JM, et al: Intravenous DSA of intracranial carotid lesions. Comparison with other techniques and specimens. AJNR 5:547–552, 1984.
48. Hesselink JR, Hayman LA, Chung KJ, et al: Myocardial ischemia during intravenous digital subtraction angiography in patients with cardiac disease. 69th Scientific Assembly and Annual Meeting, Radiol Soc North Am (Chicago). November, 1983.
49. Pinto RS, Manuell M, Kricheff II: Complications of digital intravenous angiography: Experience in 2488 cervicocranial examinations. AJNR 5:553–557, 1984.
50. Pinto RS, Seeger JF, Carmody RF: Radiologic evaluation of the carotid arteries. CRC Crit Rev Diagn Imag 22:127–162, 1984.
51. Aaron JO, Hesselink JR, Oot R, et al: Complications of intravenous DSA performed for carotid artery disease: A prospective study. Radiology 153:675–678, 1984.
52. Worthington C, Peters TM, Ethier R, et al: Stereoscopic digital subtraction angiography in neurological assessment. AJNR 6:802–808, 1985.
53. Takahashi M: Clinical usefulness of stereoscopic DSA. Appl Radiol Mar/Apr, 35–43, 1986.
54. Miller F: Tomographic DSA said to reduce motion artifacts. Diagn Imag Jan, 11, 1986.
55. Thiele BL, Young JV, Chikos PM, et al: Correlation of arteriographic findings and symptoms in cerebrovascular disease. Neurology 30:1041–1046, 1980.
56. Zwiebel WJ, Crummy AB: Sources of error in doppler diagnosis of carotid occlusive disease. AJNR 2:231–242, 1981.
57. Garth KE, Carroll BA, Sommer FG, et al: Duplex ultrasound scanning of the carotid arteries with velocity spectrum analysis. Radiology 147:823–827, 1983.
58. O'Donnell TF Jr, Erdoes L, Mackey WC, et al: Correlation of B-mode ultrasound imaging and arteriography with pathologic findings at carotid endarterectomy. Arch Surg 120:443–449, 1985.
59. Jackson VP, Kuehn DS, Bendick PJ, et al: Duplex carotid sonography: Correlation with digital subtraction angiography and conventional angiography. J Ultrasound Med 4:239–249, 1985.
60. Fischer GC, Anderson DC, Farber R, et al: Prediction of carotid disease by ultrasound and digital subtraction angiography. Arch Neurol 42:224–227, 1985.
61. Jacobs NM, Grant EG, Schellinger D, et al: Duplex carotid sonography: Criteria for stenosis, accuracy, and pitfalls. Radiology 154:385–391, 1985.
62. Quinones-Baldrich WJ, Moore WS: Asymptomatic carotid stenosis and rationale for management. Arch Neurol 42:378–382, 1985.
63. Yatsu FM, Fields WS: Asymptomatic carotid bruit, stenosis or ulceration, a conservative approach. Arch Neurol 42:383–385, 1985.
64. Hachinski V: Asymptomatic carotid bruit, stenosis or ulceration, a conservative approach (Comment). Arch Neurol 42:385, 1985.
65. Wagner ML, Singleton EB, Egan ME: Digital subtraction angiography in children. AJR 140:127–133, 1983.
66. Faerber EN, Griska LAB, Swartz JD, et al: Digital subtraction angiography in pediatric cerebrovascular occlusive disease. Radiology 152:391–394, 1984.
67. Debrun GM, Vinuela FV, Fox AJ: Aspirin and systemic heparinization in diagnostic and interventional neuroradiology. AJR 139:139–142, 1982.
68. Eriksson I, Jorulf H: Surgical complications associated with arterial catheterization. Scand J Thorac Cardiovasc Surg 4:69–75, 1970.
69. Ross RS: Cooperative study of cardiac catheterization. Arterial complications. Circulation (Suppl) 37,38:39–41, 1968.
70. Zollikofer CL, Castaneda-Zuniga WR, Galliani CA, et al: Combination of stainless steel coil and compressed Ivalon: A new technique for embolization of large arteries and arteriovenous fistulas. Radiology 138:229, 1981.

71. Dubois PJ, Kerber CW, Heinz ER: Interventional techniques in neuroradiology. Radiol Clin North Am 27:514–542, 1979.
72. Latchaw RE, Gold LHA: Polyvinyl foam embolization of vascular and neoplastic lesions of the head, neck, and spine. Radiology 131:669–679, 1979.
73. Hieshima GB, Everhart FR, Mehringer CM, et al: Preoperative embolization of meningiomas. Surg Neurol 14:119–127, 1980.
74. Ahn HS, Kerber CW, Deeb ZL: Extra- to intracranial arterial anastomoses in therapeutic embolization: Recognition and role. AJNR 1:71–75, 1980.
75. Handa J, Nakasu S, Matsuda I: Facial nerve palsy following therapeutic embolization. Surg Neurol 14:377–380, 1980.

CHAPTER 4

Outpatient Low-Dose Myelographic Techniques

Arthur B. Dublin, M.D.

Low-dose plain film myelography (LDM), alone or in combination with computed tomography (CT), may still be an appropriate tool in the evaluation of spinal disorders, even with the availability of high-resolution noncontrast CT and, more recently, magnetic resonance imaging (MRI).[1-9] The limited availability of MRI in some locations and the increased costs of inpatient studies versus outpatient examinations in conjunction with CT myelography (CTM) make LDM a significant alternative for the detection of spinal disease.[10] This discussion will describe the techniques of this latter approach to the investigation of spinal pathology and the appropriate indications for these examinations.

INDICATIONS FOR LDM/CTM AND COMPARISON WITH OTHER IMAGING MODALITIES

LDM is a technique employing reduced volumes and concentrations of water-soluble nonionic materials, either as a single procedure or, more commonly, in conjunction with CT. This technique is especially useful for improving thecal sac-disk interface contrast resolution for patients with equivocal or nondiagnostic plain CT studies (such as in postoperative or obese individuals).[6] In addition, LDM and CTM may be alternatives for individuals who feel claustrophobic with MRI. Finally, some patients may have mobile herniated disks, which can only be demonstrated by a weight-bearing position (Fig. 4–1).[6] Although newer agents such as iohexol

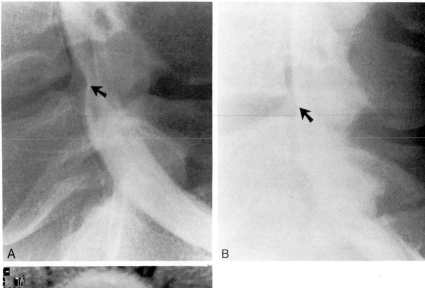

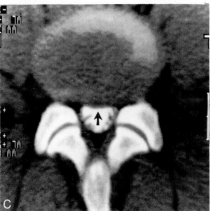

Figure 4–1. The effect of weight-bearing on a mobile herniated disk. *(A)* Lateral prone semiupright, weight-bearing, low-dose plain film myelogram. A moderately large protrusion is seen at L4–L5 (arrow). *(B)* Lateral prone, horizontal, non–weight-bearing view. In this position, the disk protrusion of L4–L5 is only faintly suggested (arrow). *(C)* The prone axial CT following *B* shows only a hint of the disk protrusion at L4–L5 (arrow).

(Omnipaque)* and iopamidol (Isovue)† appear to reduce the morbidity of myelography, these agents are not totally free of side effects.[11–15] Lowered concentrations and volumes of these materials (extrapolated from metrizamide studies) may possibly protect the patient against the side effects of headache, nausea, and vomiting.[5–9]

A prospective study by Modic and colleagues evaluated 60 patients with suspected lumbar herniated disk by surface coil MRI (0.6 tesla), CT, and/or myelography. They concluded that MRI was equivalent to CT in combination with myelography in the accuracy of detection of disk disease

---

*Winthrop-Breon, New York, NY
†Squibb Diagnostics, New Brunswick, NJ

(Figs. 4–2, 4–3, 4–4).[4] However, MRI does offer several advantages over other imaging techniques (Table 4–1), including direct multiplanar imaging, no known health effects, superiority in evaluating spinal cord disease (especially syringohydromyelia), and reduced artifacts from moderate-sized amounts of nonferromagnetic surgical implants compared with CT.[2–14, 16] However, MRI does have several distinct disadvantages, such as longer imaging times (which may allow considerable motion artifacts in uncomfortable or claustrophobic patients), a lack of weight-bearing stresses on disk spaces, and the inability to image certain groups of patients (those with pacemakers or cerebral aneurysm clips and those on respirators).[2–4] In addition, our own experience shows that a certain percentage of patients feel so severely claustrophobic as to be unable to undergo MRI examination. This drop-out effect was approximately 1 in 20 patients with our initial 0.5-tesla MRI. However, the updated 1.5 tesla unit has improved ventilation, communication, and lighting. These factors, combined with our technologists' increased experience in patient interaction, have decreased the drop-out rate to 1 in 150 examinations.[17] Finally, larger metal implants and ferromagnetic substances can cause considerable MRI image degradation.[2–4]

Plain CT is excellent for evaluating trauma and the analysis of fine bone detail.[1] However, the evaluation of degenerative disk disease, if MRI is not appropriate, is best accomplished by the combination of LDM and CTM. This combination allows flexion and extension motions to evaluate spinal stability in cases of spondylolisthesis and trauma, to place weight-bearing stresses on mobile disks to improve their detection rate, and to improve thecal sac-disk interface contrast.[6–7] Intravenous contrast has been reported as valuable in differentiating scar from recurrent disk and in improving disk-epidural space contrast (especially in the cervical region).[18–20] We have not found intravenous contrast-enhanced CT to be as reliable as described in the literature, although on occasion it may have some use in differentiating prominent epidural plexuses from disk herniation/fragmentation.[21] CTM may be inaccurate in the diagnosis of syringo-hydromyelia, since contrast may occasionally cross into the normal spinal cord or into posttraumatic myelomalacia without cavitation.[22–23] However, CTM may be more sensitive than LDM in the detection of slowly filling arachnoid cysts or intraspinal meningoceles because of the superior contrast resolution of CT (Fig. 4–5).

TECHNIQUE OF THE EXAMINATION

The patient signs a simple informed consent explaining the basic risks and benefits of the procedure. Preparation by patients includes their usual medications, good hydration with clear liquids, and accompaniment by a

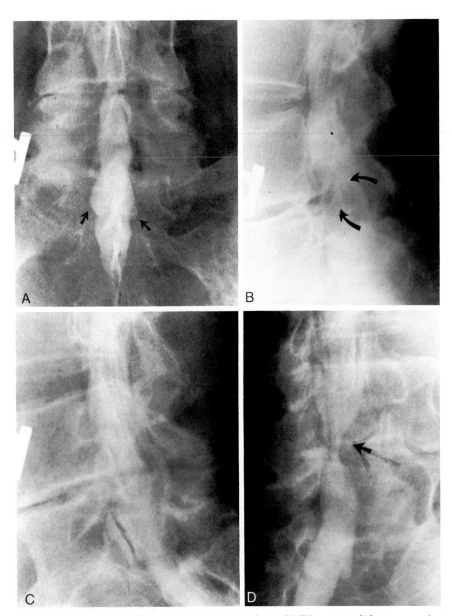

Figure 4–2. Comparison of low-dose CT myelography and MRI in a postdiskectomy patient with recurrent radiculopathy and herniated disk. *(A)* Posteroanterior, weight-bearing 100-mm spot film reveals some blunting and irregularity of the thecal sac (arrows), compatible with a moderate degree of arachnoiditis. *(B)* A lateral film shows a large defect at L4–L5 upon the thecal sac (arrows). *(C and D)* oblique views demonstrate a large right-sided extraarachnoid defect at L4–L5 (arrow).

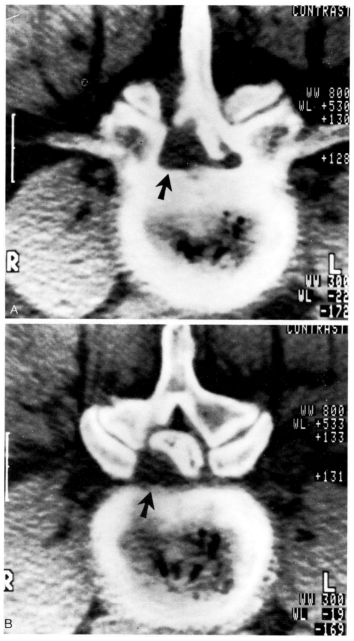

Figure 4–3. Computed tomography following the study shown in Figure 4–2. *(A and B)* Axial CT sections show a large extraarachnoid defect compatible with a recurrent herniated disk (arrows).

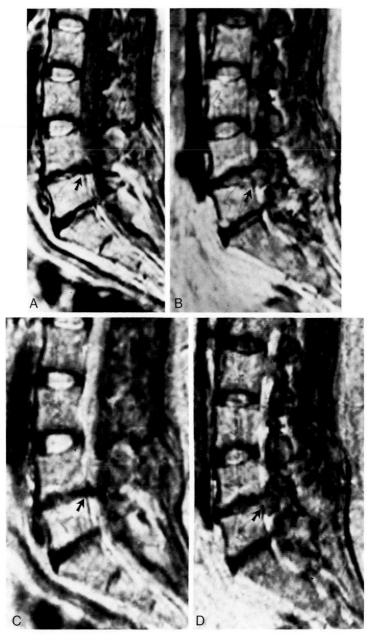

Figure 4–4. Sagittal MRI of the same patient as Figure 4–2, with mild motion artifacts. (*A* and *B*) Spin echo, 1350/50, first echo, 7-mm sections, 0.5 tesla shows a large rounded mass of medium signal intensity to the right of midline, compatible with a herniated disk (arrows). (*C* and *D*) Second echo, more T2-weighted images again show the herniated disk (arrows).

Table 4–1
LDM/CTM VERSUS PLAIN CT OR MRI

	LDM/CTM	Plain CT	MRI
Complications due to contrast/spinal needle	Present	Absent	Absent
Thecal sac-disk interphase	Good	Variable	Excellent
Poor exam due to claustrophobia	Rare	Rare	1–5%
Poor exam due to exam time and back pain	Unusual	Unusual	5–15%
Weight-bearing present during exam	Present (LDM)	Absent	Absent
Flexion/extension stresses	Present (LDM)	Special views (limited)	Present (limited)

CT, computed tomography; LDM/CTM, low-dose myelography in conjunction with CT; MRI, magnetic resonance imaging.

responsible adult to drive them home after the examination. No intravenous line is usually started, except to administer intravenous sedation for extremely anxious patients. Diazepam (Valium),* 5 mg PO 30 minutes before the study, is an alternative for moderately anxious patients or for individuals with muscle spasm. However, most patients need no premedication.

After appropriate sterile preparation and local anesthesia of the back, the patient is placed on his or her stomach, the head is elevated 20 degrees, and a 25-gauge needle is introduced into the L2–L3 interspace. There is evidence to suggest that a smaller needle size is related to a decreased incidence of side effects.[7, 24-25] In addition, a 20-gauge needle is easier to steer through narrow openings between the posterior elements affected by osteophytic disease, especially in elderly patients. A midline approach is usually satisfactory, although an off-midline technique may be desired in individuals with severe hypertrophic spurring.

Five to 7 ml of iohexol (100 mg iodine/ml concentration) or a similar agent, coupled with 100-mm fluoroscopic and occasional standard filming techniques, provides an excellent detailed study of the low back. The routine removal of cerebrospinal fluid (CSF) is not appropriate or productive, and CSF analysis should therefore be directed by the clinical circumstances.[26] Upright 100-mm spot films (with lateral flexion/extension), anteroposterior, and oblique views are obtained (Fig. 4–6). A conventional cross-table lateral film is taken with the patient in a non–weight-bearing prone position to visualize better the upper lumbar region. Digital subtraction and myelographic techniques of cooperative individuals may be useful to decrease the effects of superimposed osseous structures and to improve contrast resolution with acceptable spatial resolution (Fig. 4–7).[27-28]

---

*Roche Laboratories, Nutley, NJ

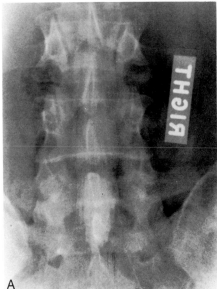

Figure 4–5. (A) Posteroanterior early film demonstrates nonfilling of an intrasacral arachnoid cyst. (B and C) The contrast is seen in the thecal sac (straight arrows) and in the arachnoid cyst (curved arrows).

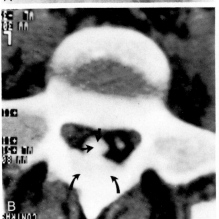

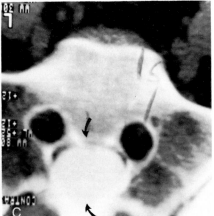

Slightly higher volumes and concentrations (7 to 10 ml of iohexol [150 mg iodine/ml concentration]) are suitable for the examination of the cervical and thoracic spine, via a lumbar puncture route. In general, the cervical puncture technique is more uncomfortable for the patient than is the lumbar approach. In addition, the former procedure poses more of a danger of significant needle-related complications. The lumbar approach is therefore preferred at our facility for neck examinations.[29–31]

The side effects of nausea and vomiting may be the same whether the patient is ambulated or kept at bed rest.[32–33] These side effects are also probably unchanged with cervical myelography performed via the cervical

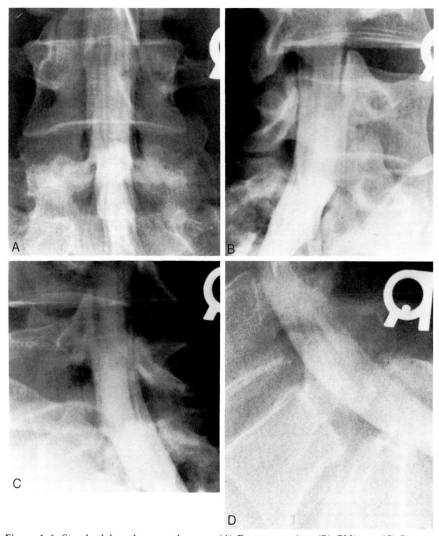

Figure 4–6. Standard low-dose myelogram. *(A)* Posteroanterior. *(B)* Oblique. *(C)* Reverse oblique. *(D)* Neutral.

Illustration continued on following page

or lumbar puncture route, although the amount of contrast found within the skull and the electroencephalographic (EEG) abnormalities observed were increased with the cervical technique.[34]

Following the plain film examination, the patient is transported in a supine position to the CT scanner, placed prone, and appropriate angled and nonangled sections are taken at 3- or 4.5-mm intervals and slice thicknesses, depending on whether the cervical or lumbothoracic region

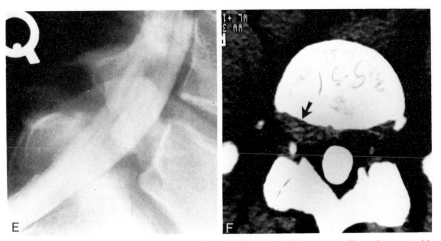

Figure 4–6 *Continued (E)* Flexion semiupright weight-bearing 100-mm spot films show a stable first-degree spondylolisthesis of L5–S1. *(F)* A selected axial CT view of L5–S1 shows a small right-sided disk herniation (arrow), not demonstrated by the plain radiographs.

is examined, respectively. The prone technique facilitates abutment of the contrast agent against the disk spaces. With dilutions of contrast as prescribed above, additional rotation of the patient to promote mixing of contrast is generally not needed. A typical lumbar study will include L3–S1, plus several 12-mm sections of the conus region. Reformations, using multiple 1- to 2-mm axial slice thicknesses, may be of some limited use in the evaluation of lateral foraminal osteophytic disease, fractures, and spondylotic defects, although in our experience such techniques are not otherwise particularly helpful.[35]

The patient is then placed in the slightly head-up supine position and observed for 1 hour. Although the study by Kostiner and Krook suggests that bed rest may be too conservative an approach and that ambulation at home without bed rest may be an acceptable alternative to recumbency, other authors suggest bed rest with head elevation for 24 hours.[5–10, 32] Most patients have back discomfort that is best relieved by a non–weight-bearing position.[32] The patient is then driven home by a companion and instructed to remain recumbent with the head elevated on two pillows (to facilitate gradual dilution and absorption of the contrast medium), with bathroom privileges for the remainder of the day. No alcoholic or caffeinated drinks are allowed (these will promote diuresis), but other fluids are encouraged. A contact 24-hour telephone number is given to the patient in case problems arise.

COMPLICATIONS

Cognitive changes and somatic side effects have been evaluated after the introduction of metrizamide and newer nonionic agents.[11–15] Ratcliff and

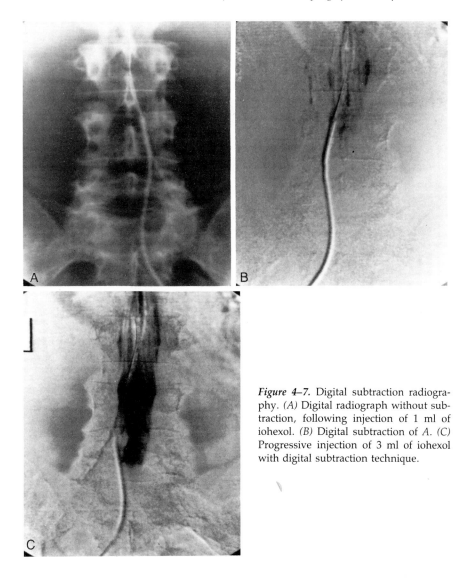

Figure 4–7. Digital subtraction radiography. *(A)* Digital radiograph without subtraction, following injection of 1 ml of iohexol. *(B)* Digital subtraction of *A*. *(C)* Progressive injection of 3 ml of iohexol with digital subtraction technique.

colleagues suggest that metrizamide produces greater mood and cognitive functional changes than iohexol, if 300 mg/ml of iodine concentration or both agents are introduced via a C1–C2 puncture route for cervical myelography.[14] In addition, Hammeke and associates suggest that iopamidol produces fewer somatic side effects than metrizamide.[15] Similar differences in headache, nausea, and vomiting are also intensified.[11–13] Witwer and colleagues found that iopamidol was also less toxic than metrizamide when both agents were used in concentrations of 200 to 300 mg of iodine/ml in the examination of the lumbar and cervical spine (the latter via a C1–C2 puncture).[1]

The use of iophendylater (Pantopaque)* for cervical myelography was still widespread in the United States as late as 1983, as suggested by the results of a survey conducted by Dublin.[36] This was probably due in part to the greater ease of maneuverability of iophendylate and the decreased side effects of seizure and hallucination, as compared with water-soluble agents. However, iophendylate has several serious drawbacks, as compared with water-soluble agents: (1) the production of severe artifacts when CT is used as an adjunct to plain film myelography, (2) the production of a pseudolipoma appearance of MRI, (3) the need for removal of iophendylate following the filming sequence, (4) the suggestion by some studies that iophendylate may lead to increased CSF pleocytosis and arachnoiditis, especially if contaminated by talc glove powder, and (5) the increased difficulty in passing iophendylate past regions of almost total CSF blockade by pathologies.[3-4, 37-39] Iophendylate does give a "denser" filling of the CSF, is easier to maneuver from the lumbar to the cervical regions, does not have the seizure potential of metrizamide, and is less expensive than water-soluble preparations. However, the overall advantages of less-toxic agents such as iohexol and iopamidol suggest that these newer preparations should be used preferentially and should form the basis for the standard of quality of care for myelography.

Many facilities still use the direct cervical puncture technique for performing cervical myelography.[36] However, the side effects of direct needle trauma to the spinal cord and to the adjacent vasculature can be significant.[29-31] Furthermore, the cervical approach may be more painful than the lumbar technique, partly because of the natural reluctance of the examiner to place local anesthesia deeply into the neck for fear of injecting

---

*Lafayette Pharmacal, Inc, Lafayette, Indiana

Table 4–2
COMPLICATIONS OF OUTPATIENT MYELOGRAPHY
USING METRIZAMIDE

Authors	Volume (ml)	Concentration (mg Iodine/ml)	Needle Size	Asymptomatic Patients
Zinreich[9]	?	100	25	72/80 (90%)
Zinreich[9]	5	170	22	16/25 (64%)
Tate*[8]	5–10	180	25	38/79 (48%)
Kostinger*[32]	13–18	190	22	22/70 (31%)
Dublin[6]	3.5	150	25	6/10 (60%)
Dublin[7]	5	110	25	41/45 (91%)
Pressman[5]	2.5	170	22/25	20/40 (50%)
Badani[10]	4–13	200	22	48/228 (25%)

*2–3 ml CSF removed before contrast agent injected.

xylocaine into the spinal cord or thecal sac. The advent of superior fluoroscopic spot devices, special patient positioning (such as the oblique lateral position for very kyphotic individuals), and the judicial use of digital techniques allow the examiner to use dilute quantities of water-soluble contrast agents, via a lumbar puncture, to obtain high-quality examinations of the neck and upper thoracic spine.[40]

Table 4–2 suggests that dilute and reduced quantities of metrizamide reduce the degree of side effects produced by myelography, as compared with full-dose metrizamide techniques. A controlled study using identical needle sizes, approaches, and postrecovery procedures, with both full- and low-strength newer agents such as iopamidol and iohexol, has not to my knowledge been undertaken. Since these agents are not totally free of side effects, however, it is not unreasonable to expect that reduced concentrations (such as those used in our current protocol) will produce fewer adverse reactions.

COST-EFFECTIVENESS OF OUTPATIENT LOW-DOSE MYELOGRAPHY

Badami and colleagues suggested that outpatient metrizamide myelography could be performed safely and with significant cost savings.[10] He calculated a 20% reduction in cost by using the outpatient technique, or $110,000 per year for 800 myelograms. Our own calculations show a total

Table 4–3
FLOW PATTERN USED IN CHOOSING
IMAGING MODALITIES

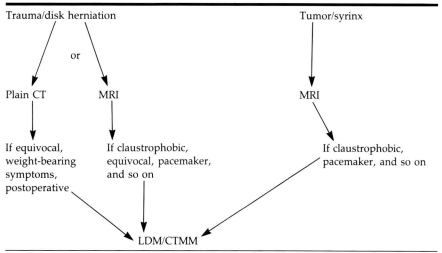

cost (including technical and professional fees) of $770 for the plain film myelogram and the postmyelographic CT. This charge is all-inclusive, including the postrecovery time. We have found that our price is approximately 10% less than the typical combined inpatient professional and technical charge for our area. In addition, the overnight semiprivate room expense, not including any extras such as medications, is approximately $350. Thus, the typical total hospital bill for this examination may total almost $1,200 per patient. Our projected cost savings for every 800 patients undergoing *outpatient* CTM is therefore over $350,000. The amount of money saved depends on many factors, but the important message is that outpatient studies of this type are cost-effective and safe.

CONCLUSION

Outpatient LDM techniques, especially in combination with CT, may be cost-effective, appropriate measures and complement MRI examinations. Table 4–3 outlines a flow pattern that is useful in choosing between the different modalities.

References

1. Newton TH, Potts DG (eds): Computed Tomography of the Spine and Spinal Cord. Modern Neuroradiology. San Anselmo, Clavadel Press, 1983.
2. Paushter DM, Modic MI, Masaryk TJ: Magnetic resonance imaging of the spine: Applications and limitations. Radiol Clin North Am 23:551–562, 1985.
3. Modic MT, Masaryk T, Paushter D: Magnetic resonance imaging of the spine. Radiol Clin North Am 24:229–245, 1986.
4. Modic MT, Masaryk T, Boumphrey F, et al: Lumbar herniated disk disease and canal stenosis: Prospective evaluation by surface coil MR, CT, and myelography. AJR 147:757–765, 1986.
5. Pressman BD, Mink JH, Turner RM, et al: Low-dose metrizamide spinal computed tomography in outpatients. J Comput Assist Tomogr 10:817–821, 1986.
6. Dublin AB, McGahan JP, Reid MH: The value of computed tomographic metrizamide myelography in the neurological evaluation of the spine. Radiology 146:79–86, 1983.
7. Dublin AB, Reid MH: Outpatient low-dose computed tomography metrizamide myelography and evaluation of lumbar disk disease. CT J Comput Tomogr 8:113–117, 1984.
8. Tate CF III, Wilkov HR, Lestrange NK, et al: Outpatient lumbar myelography. Initial results in 79 examinations using a low-dose metrizamide technique. Radiology 157:391–393, 1985.
9. Zinreich SJ, Wang H, Updike ML, et al: CT myelography for outpatients: An inpatient/outpatient pilot study to assess methodology. Radiology 157:387–390, 1985.
10. Badami JP, Baker RA, Scholz FJ, et al: Outpatient metrizamide myelography: Prospective evaluation of safety and cost-effectiveness. Radiology 158:175–177, 1986.
11. Witwer G, Cacayorin ED, Berstein AD, et al: Iopamidol and metrizamide for myelography: Prospective double-blind clinical trial. AJNR 5:403–407, 1984.
12. Gebarski SS, Gabrielsen TO, Knake JE, et al: Iohexol versus metrizamide for cervical myelography: Double-blind trial. AJNR 6:923–926, 1985.

13. Latchaw RE, Hirsch WL, Horton JA, et al: Iohexol versus metrizamide: A study of efficacy and morbidity in cervical myelography. AJNR 6:931–933, 1985.
14. Ratcliff G, Sandler S, Latchaw R: Cognitive and effective changes after myelography: A comparison of metrizamide and iohexol. AJR 147:777–781, 1986.
15. Hammeke TA, Grogan JP, Haughton VM: Evaluation of myelographic contrast-medium tolerance with psychometric testing. AJNR 6:343–348, 1985.
16. Shellock FG: Biological effects of MRI: A clear safety record so far. Diagn Imag 9:96–101, 1987.
17. Hess TP: Skills of technologists can make or break an MRI center. Diagn Imag 9:85–93, 1987.
18. Russell EJ, D'Angelo CM, Zimmerman RD, et al: Cervical disk herniation: CT demonstration after contrast enhancement. Radiology 152:703–712, 1984.
19. Teplick JB, Haskin ME: Intravenous contrast-enhanced CT of the postoperative lumbar spine: Improved identification of recurrent disk herniation, scar, arachnoiditis, and diskitis. AJNR 5:373–383, 1984.
20. Braun IF, Hoffman JC Jr, Davis PC, et al: Contrast enhancement in CT differentiation between recurrent disk herniation and postoperative scar: Prospective study. AJNR 6:607–612, 1985.
21. Reid MH, Dublin AB: Epidural venography during computed tomography of the spine. Int Soc Radiol Annu Meet (Brussels), 1981.
22. Cooper PR, Cohen W: Evaluation of cervical spinal cord injuries with metrizamide myelography-CT scanning. J Neurosurg 61:281–289, 1984.
23. Iwasaki Y, Abe H, Isu T, et al: CT myelography with intramedullary enhancement in cervical spondylosis. J Neurosurg 63:363–366, 1985.
24. Sinclaire D, Ritchie G: Morbidity and post-myelogram patients: A survey of 100 patients. J Can Assoc Radiol 23:278–283, 1972.
25. Toyrtellotte W, Henderson W, Tucker R: A randomized, double-blind clinical trial comparing the .22 versus .26 gauge needle in the production of the post lumbar puncture syndrome in normal individuals. Headache 12:23, 1972.
26. Rothfus WE, Latchaw RE: Nonefficacy of routine removal of CSF during neurodiagnostic procedures. AJNR 5:797–800, 1984.
27. Tsai FY, Hieshima G, Mellor R, et al: Digital metrizamide myelography. West Neuroradiol Soc (Napa), 1983.
28. Sherry RE, Anderson RE: Real-time digitally subtracted fluoroscopy for cervical myelography. Radiology 15:243–248, 1988.
29. Johansen JB, Orrison WW, Amundsen P: Lateral C1–C2 puncture for cervical myelography. Part I. Report of a complication. Radiology 146:391–393, 1983.
30. Orrison WW, Edevik OP, Sackett JF: Lateral C1–C2 puncture for cervical myelography. Part II. Recognition of improper injection of contrast material. Radiology 146:395–400, 1983.
31. Orrison WW, Edevik OP, Sackett JF: Lateral C1–C2 puncture for cervical myelography. Part III. Historical, anatomic, and technical considerations. Radiology 146:401–408, 1983.
32. Kostiner AI, Krook PM: Outpatient lumbar myelography with metrizamide. Radiology 155:383–385, 1985.
33. Teasdale E, MacPherson P: Incidence of side effects following direct puncture cervical myelography. Neuroradiology 25:85–86, 1983.
34. MacPherson P, Teasdale E, McGeorge AP: Direct puncture versus run up cervical myelography with iopamidol: A comparison of side effects, EEG changes, and radiographic quality. J Neurol Neurosurg Psychiatry 46:959–962, 1983.
35. Rothman SLG, Glenn WV Jr: CT multiplanar in 253 cases of lumbar spondylosis. AJNR 5:81–90, 1984.
36. Dublin AB: An analysis of current radiological practice in the evaluation of disorders of the spine. West Neuroradiol Soc (Napa), 1983.

37. Haughton VM, Ho K-C: Arachnoid response to contrast media: A comparison of iophendylate and metrizamide in experimental animals. Radiology 143:699–702, 1982.
38. Johansen JB, Bartholemy CR, Haughton VM, et al: Arachnoiditis from myelography and laminectomy in experimental animals. AJNR 5:97–99, 1984.
39. Khan A, Marc JA, Chen M, et al: Total myelography with metrizamide through the lumbar route. AJR 136:771–776, 1981.
40. Williams AG, Seigel RS, Kornfeld M, et al: Experimental production of arachnoiditis with glove powder contamination during myelography. AJNR 3:121–125, 1982.

CHAPTER 5

Interventional Procedures for the Breast

Karen K. Lindfors, M.D., and
Daniel B. Kopans, M.D.

Aggressive mammographic screening programs have been shown to re-duce mortality from breast cancer. In order to be effective, however, a screening program must be affiliated with a center where interventional procedures for the breast are readily available. Needle localizations of occult breast lesions, cyst aspirations, and needle aspiration biopsies are important in diagnosing the exact nature of abnormalities found on mammographic examinations. All of these interventional procedures can be performed easily on an outpatient basis. No particular patient prepa-ration is necessary for these procedures, except when a biopsy is to follow a localization. In these cases, the routine preoperative instructions of the surgeon or anesthesiologist will be followed by the patient.

LOCALIZATION OF OCCULT BREAST LESIONS

As the demand for mammography grows, so does the demand for accurate preoperative localization of suspicious but clinically occult breast lesions. Many methods for localization of nonpalpable lesions have been described. In choosing a technique, the radiologist should decide which method will allow sufficient accuracy so that only small volumes of tissue are removed at biopsy. Since malignancies will be found in only 10 to 24% of all biopsies performed for suspicious mammographic abnormalities, and therefore more than 75% of all lesions biopsied will be benign, accurate excision with preservation of as much normal tissue as possible should be the goal of any localization and biopsy.[1, 2]

In most patients, mammographically guided localizations and subsequent biopsies of occult breast lesions can be performed on an outpatient basis. The patient should arrive in the radiology department 1 to 2 hours prior to her scheduled time in the operating room. Since most localizations require a seated, cooperative patient, sedation should be omitted.

If craniocaudal and lateral projections are available from a recent previous study, no preliminary mammograms are necessary. If only a previous oblique view is available, however, a straight lateral view should be taken before the localization procedure begins to triangulate better the position of the lesion in the breast.

To decide which approach should be used, the radiologist should determine which skin surface of the breast is closest to the lesion and then use that surface as a point of entry. Either the craniocaudal, mediolateral, or lateromedial approach may be used. The caudacranial approach can be used to approach inferior lesions if the tube will swing 180 degrees. This latter technique may be awkward for the radiologist, however, and in most cases the next closest skin surface will be used to approach inferior lesions. The patient should then be placed in the position that will allow the radiologist access to the skin surface closest to the lesion.

Most currently available dedicated film-screen mammographic units are equipped with guidance systems that facilitate accurate positioning of localizing needles. Such systems allow placement of needles in a position parallel to the chest wall. In so doing, complications that may be associated with positioning a needle directed toward the chest wall, such as transgression of the pleura or placement of a hook-wire into the pectoralis muscles, can be avoided. A similar approach is suggested and can be used when localizations are performed with xerographic guidance.

At this point there is some divergence in localization technique between a film-screen unit with rigid compression and one that will be used with xerography. The technique for film-screen guidance will be described first, and then the modifications required for use of xerography will be discussed.

Technique for Localization With Film-Screen Mammographic Units

The breast is compressed in the position determined by the radiologist from the preliminary films, as described above. A fenestrated compression plate designed specifically for localizations is used. After the film is developed, with the breast remaining in the compressed position, the coordinates of the lesion are plotted (Fig. 5–1*A*). The skin is treated with povidone-iodine (Betadine) solution, and the localizing needle is inserted perpendicular to the skin and parallel to the x-ray beam, with an effort to pass the needle through or alongside the area in question. A film is taken to ensure proper needle position in this axis and then, without movement of the patient, it is developed (Fig. 5–1*B*). The mammographic system must permit the removal of the cassette without moving the breast or releasing compression, so that the needle can be accurately repositioned if necessary.

Once the needle is positioned appropriately in the first projection, compression is slowly released and the breast tissue is pulled up around the needle. This ensures that the tip of the needle remains beyond the lesion so that even if there is movement of the breast, the lesion will remain on the shaft of the needle. The patient is then moved away from the unit and the tube is rotated 90 degrees so the x-ray beam is perpendicular to the shaft of the needle. A spot compression device is then placed over the shaft of the needle and positioned so that the lesion and the needle tip can be seen on the film (Fig. 5–1*C*). The standard collimator is used so that some of the surrounding uncompressed tissue can be seen in order to provide landmarks if further repositioning is required. With the spot compression device there is complete access to the hub of the needle, and after a film is taken to determine the depth of the needle with respect to the area of concern, the position of the needle tip can be adjusted so that it terminates in or just beyond the lesion. If a hook-wire system is to be used, the wire can then be placed through the hub of the needle, advancing it to the point where the wire exits the needle tip. At this point, the needle is withdrawn over the wire, taking care not to move the wire until the hooked end is engaged.

Once the wire is in place, a final film should be taken in the same projection to ascertain the depth of the hook-wire with respect to the lesion (Fig. 5–1*D*). The initial passage of the needle through the lesion guarantees the position of the wire in the first projection, so a film in this projection need not be repeated. The breast is allowed to assume its normal position. The portion of the wire external to the patient's skin is then loosely taped to the skin with sterile strips for the patient's comfort, and she is taken to the operating room.

Surgeons are not obligated to follow the localizing wire in their dissection. They can triangulate the position of the lesion and the localizer and use whatever approach they prefer. A stiffening cannula or a needle passed over the wire in the operating room may facilitate palpation of the localizer.

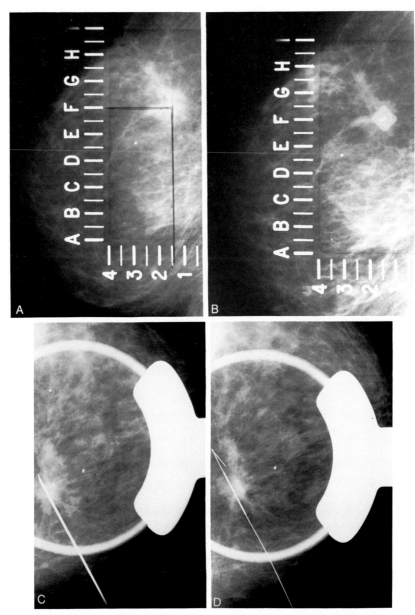

Figure 5–1. *(A)* Medial lateral mammogram using fenestrated compression plate with opening placed over the area of the lesion. Coordinates of the lesion are plotted on the film. *(B)* Localizing needle is inserted into the breast parallel to the direction of the x-ray beam and deep enough to traverse the lesion. *(C)* Craniocaudal view of the breast using spot compression perpendicular to the needle showing depth of the needle tip with respect to the lesion. *(D)* Final film taken after the hook-wire has been placed through the needle and the needle removed.

Modifications of Localization Technique for Use With Xerography

The principles of the localization method using xerography are basically the same as those used when film-screen units are employed to guide the procedures. The technique is slightly different, however, as compression is usually not necessary because of the wide exposure latitude of xeroradiography. A system by which the cassettes can be removed without moving the patient is still essential. Shelves for the cassettes can be built to fit under the surface on which the breast is positioned. Negative mode is always used to avoid artifacts that may obscure the lesion.

The initial position of the patient is determined from the preliminary films (Fig. 5–2A,B). An aluminum marker is then placed over the lesion, and a film is taken (Fig. 5–2C). The patient is instructed not to move while the film is developed. The point of entry of the needle can be adjusted using the marker as a reference. The skin is prepared, and the needle is introduced parallel to the x-ray beam (Fig. 5–2D). Once again the needle should be passed through or alongside the lesion to a point beyond the lesion, and a film is taken to assure the position of the needle. If the position is satisfactory, the patient is then carefully moved to the position that is 90 degrees opposite to that filmed initially. A picture is taken to determine the depth of the needle with respect to the area to be biopsied (Fig. 5–2E). Compression may be used if desired. Once the needle tip is adjusted to its optimal position, the hook-wire can be afterloaded and engaged as described above. A final film should then be taken (Fig. 5–2F), and the patient is transported to the operating room.

Localizing Systems

A multitude of localizing systems for occult breast lesions have been described. The first of these included such noninvasive procedures as skin markers over the lesion and stereomammography.[3, 4] Lesions were sometimes difficult to retrieve using these methods, so more invasive methods were designed. In the late 1970s, the injection of a mixture of dye through a needle inserted in the lesion was popular.[5] This is still a localization method favored by some surgeons. If there is a delay between the time of injection of dye and surgery, however, there can be diffusion of dye through the tissues, resulting in a biopsy specimen that may be larger than necessary.

The simplest method of localization is the placement of a 22-gauge needle through the lesion, but such needles may become dislodged or retracted during transport of the patient to the operating room. This problem is obviated by the use of several commercially available hook-

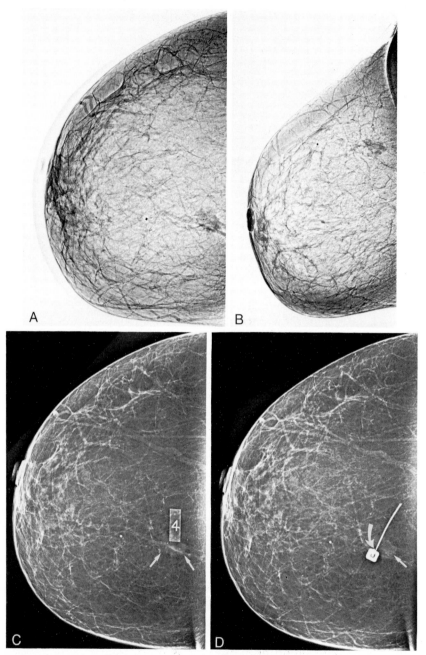

Figure 5–2. Craniocaudal *(A)* and lateral medial *(B)* positive-mode xerograms demonstrate a clinically occult suspicious mass in the upper inner aspect of the breast. *(C)* Negative-mode craniocaudal xerogram with skin marker placed just lateral to lesion (arrows). *(D)* Negative-mode craniocaudal xerogram showing needle tip (curved arrow) passing along anterior edge of lesion (straight arrow). Hook-wire remains in the needle shaft but is not engaged.

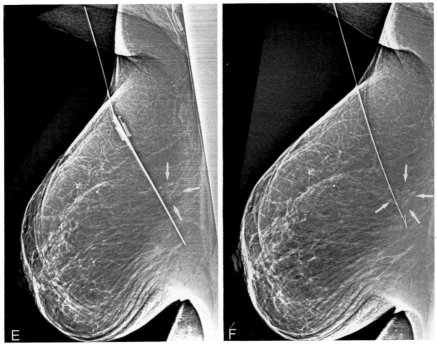

Figure 5–2 *Continued (E)* Negative-mode medial lateral xerogram showing needle passing along anterior edge of lesion (arrows). Tip of needle is located 4 cm beyond the lesion. *(F)* Final xerogram after needle was retracted and hook-wire engaged. Wire passes along anterior edge of lesion (arrows), and hook tip is located 2 cm beyond center of lesion.

wire systems that allow placement of a wire through a 20-gauge localizing needle.[6–8] These wires are "hooked" into the breast parenchyma and will not move with normal activity. Surgeons should, however, be instructed not to use the wire as a retractor but rather as a guide to the location of the lesion.

Specimen Radiography

Specimen radiography is an extremely important part of the localization and biopsy process that should not be overlooked. All specimens thought to contain calcifications or masses should be brought to the radiology department while the patient is still on the operating table. They should be wrapped in plastic wrap or put in a plastic bag and placed on the cassette border for filming. Compression of the specimen is necessary for accurate evaluation, as overlying parenchyma or trapped air might otherwise obscure the lesion. If there are several pieces of tissue, identification of the one containing the mammographic abnormality will be helpful to the pathologist.

FOLLOW-UP

All pathology reports of biopsies preceded by localization in the mammographic suite should be reviewed by the radiologist. If calcifications are removed and not seen microscopically by the pathologist or if an obviously malignant lesion was removed and a benign diagnosis made, the studies should be reviewed to assure that the appropriate lesion was examined by the pathologist. In some cases, it may be helpful to radiograph the fixed tissue to direct the pathologist toward a suspicious area.

Communication between the radiologist, surgeon, and pathologist is essential to optimal care of the patient with a suspicious clinically occult breast abnormality. A well-executed needle localization is of no value if the surgeon does not understand which area is to be removed and its relationship to the localizing device. In turn, a localization with removal of the appropriate suspicious area is not adequate if the suspicious abnormality is not examined by the pathologist.

PITFALLS

A breast lesion that can be seen in only one mammographic view presents a specific problem when it is to be localized. Such a situation can occur when the lesion is too close to the chest wall to be imaged in one position (usually the craniocaudal) or when the lesion is obscured by dense parenchyma in one view. Although these occurrences are rare, a few comments concerning the approach to localizing such lesions are necessary.

In departments where mammography is performed with a tube that moves independently of the cassette, localizations can be performed for lesions seen in only one view using the method described by Yagan and colleagues.[9] This method makes use of the geometry of the x-ray beam when it is angled and allows triangulation of lesions seen in one view. The method as described is particularly suited to xerography.

Computed tomography (CT) or ultrasonography may also be useful in needle guidance, but microcalcifications cannot usually be visualized by either of these modalities. CT is particularly useful for lesions close to the chest wall that are seen only in lateral or oblique projections (Fig. 5–3A–C). The patient is scanned supine, with her arms overhead; 5-mm slice width sections are used, and the approximate location of the lesion in the breast is determined from the mammogram in an effort to limit

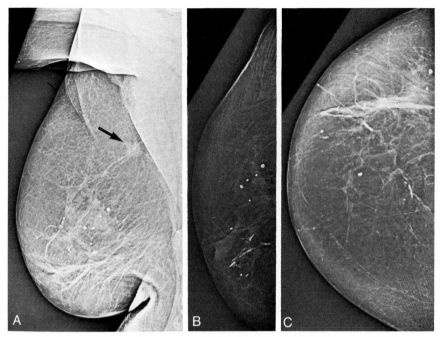

Figure 5–3. Medial lateral *(A)* negative-mode xerogram demonstrates a clinically occult suspicious mass deep in the superior portion of the breast (arrow). The mass is not visualized on either lateral *(B)* or medial *(C)* exaggerated craniocaudal views.

Illustration continued on following page

radiation exposure. An N-shaped skin marker can be taped to the skin and used to determine the exact point of entry in the skin above the lesion.[10] The depth from the skin to the lesion can be measured on CT (Fig. 5–3D). The 20-gauge needle from the localizing wire system can be inserted into the lesion and its position checked by CT (Fig. 5–3E); if the position is satisfactory, the hook-wire can then be engaged.

Sonography is most useful in guiding the aspiration of cystic lesions, but when solid masses are clearly distinguishable from the surrounding parenchyma, sonography can guide localizations. The technique used is the same as that for aspirations (described later in this chapter), except that when the needle is positioned in the lesion the hook-wire is afterloaded and engaged in the breast tissue. A final mammogram is then usually taken to determine the exact depth of the tip of the hook relative to the lesion. This technique is also particularly useful if aspiration of a lesion that is indeterminate by sonography is attempted and no fluid is obtained. The assumption is that the lesion is solid, and if previous arrangements have been made with the surgeon, a hook-wire can be afterloaded through the aspirating needle.[11]

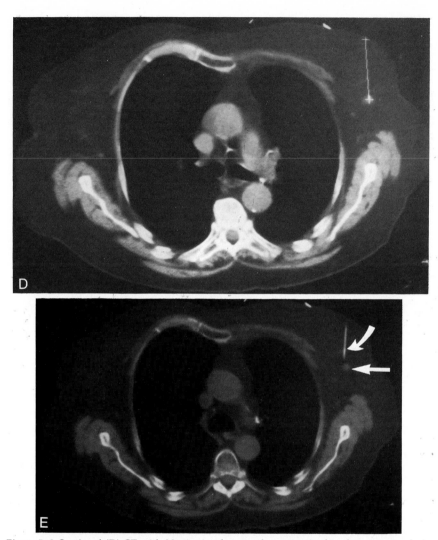

Figure 5–3 *Continued (D)* CT with N-wire in place on the patient's skin demonstrates lesion to be in the lateral aspect of the breast. Depth from the skin to the lesion is measured. *(E)* CT demonstrates 20-gauge needle (curved arrow) terminating just anterior to breast lesion (straight arrow). The needle was advanced and the hook-wire afterloaded and engaged.

TECHNIQUE FOR SONOGRAPHICALLY GUIDED CYST ASPIRATION

The breast parenchyma in the area of the lesion is flattened as much as possible by positioning the patient supine on the ultrasonography table with her ipsilateral arm placed overhead. The patient can also be placed oblique in order to flatten the parenchyma in the area for examination. A high-frequency (7.5 to 10 mHz) transducer can be used to examine the area of concern (Fig. 5–4A,B).

When the lesion to be aspirated is located, a flat plastic tube (coffee stirrer) can be positioned between the transducer and the skin, and the shadow of the device can be used to determine a skin point above the lesion (Fig. 5–4C). After the point of entry is determined, the patient should not move. The skin is prepared with povidone-iodine, and a 20-gauge needle with connecting tubing and a syringe attached is inserted into the lesion. It is helpful to have an assistant to aspirate while the needle is located in the cyst so that the position can be maintained. The disposition of the fluid obtained is controversial. Some experts believe that all fluid should be sent for cytologic analysis because of the small risk of intracystic carcinoma.

After the aspirating needle is removed, firm pressure is applied in an attempt to prevent hematoma or reaccumulation of fluid within the cyst. Follow-up sonography of the area is then performed to detect any residual fluid,[11] and a mammogram is taken to confirm complete resolution of the lesion (Fig. 5–4D,E).

Many palpable cysts are aspirated in the clinician's office, thus allowing a rapid diagnosis and obviating the need for sonography. Cysts may be difficult to penetrate because of thick fibrous walls or may be mobile enough to roll away from the aspirating needle. If aspiration of such a clinically apparent cyst fails, sonography may be of assistance in distinguishing cystic from solid masses and in performing a guided aspiration and avoiding open biopsy of a cyst.

Sonographically guided aspiration can also be of help in assessing the lesion that is indeterminate by sonography. As stated previously, if fluid is not obtained, a localizing wire can be afterloaded through the aspiration needle and the patient can proceed to open biopsy.

TECHNIQUE FOR MAMMOGRAPHICALLY GUIDED CYST ASPIRATION

Cyst aspirations can also be guided by mammography using a technique similar to that employed for needle localizations. The fenestrated compression plate is placed over the lesion, and the coordinates of the cyst are plotted on the preliminary film (Fig. 5–5A). A 19-gauge needle is inserted into the cyst in a direction parallel to the x-ray beam. When the lesion is entered, fluid will usually flow out of the needle hub (Fig. 5–5B) as a result of breast compression. The cyst should then be totally aspirated, and a postaspiration mammogram should be obtained to confirm resolution of the lesion (Fig. 5–5C). Most cysts that are aspirated using mam-

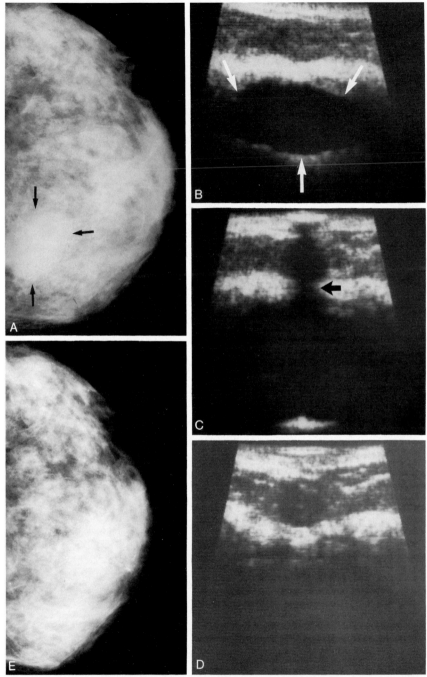

Figure 5–4. *(A)* Craniocaudal mammogram demonstrating a 4-cm mass medially (arrows). *(B)* Ultrasonography demonstrates that the lesion is probably cystic (arrows). *(C)* A flat plastic tube (coffee stirrer) is placed over the lesion between the skin and the transducer. Note the shadow cast by the device (arrow). *(D and E)* Postaspiration ultrasonography *(D)* demonstrates total resolution of the cyst, as does the postaspiration mammogram *(E).*

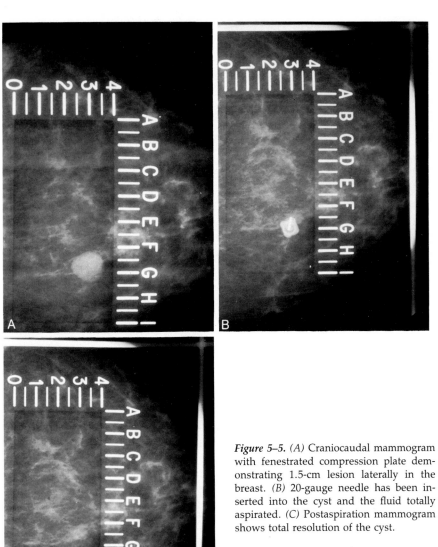

Figure 5–5. (A) Craniocaudal mammogram with fenestrated compression plate demonstrating 1.5-cm lesion laterally in the breast. (B) 20-gauge needle has been inserted into the cyst and the fluid totally aspirated. (C) Postaspiration mammogram shows total resolution of the cyst.

mographic guidance will be in patients who are referred for localizations and in whom the cystic nature of the lesion is not known prior to the procedure. In these cases, aspiration can be accomplished through the 20-gauge needle of the localizing system if the hook-wire has been removed. If the cyst can be totally aspirated and the fluid composition does not suggest old blood, subsequent biopsy is unnecessary.

NEEDLE ASPIRATION BIOPSIES

Fine-needle aspiration biopsy (FNAB) has become a helpful tool in the preoperative evaluation of suspicious palpable breast masses. It is a cost-effective technique that can avoid the need for biopsy and aid preoperative planning. The specificity of FNAB diagnosis is reported to be between 96 and 100%. Sensitivity of the procedure is somewhat lower, at 65 to 89%.[12–15] Such aspirations are generally performed by the clinician or a cytologist using a 23-gauge needle attached to a 5-ml syringe, with continuous suction applied while several passages through the lesion are made.

FNAB of nonpalpable breast lesions has not been used extensively in this country but has been successful in one reported Swedish study.[16] A fenestrated compression plate with localizing capabilities similar to that used for needle localizations was used to guide biopsies of occult lesions. Diagnostic material was obtained in 73% of cases, and all lesions were 2 cm or less in size. The sensitivity and the specificity of FNAB in this study were similar to those reported for palpable lesions in cases in which adequate tissue was obtained. Follow-up of this group of patients for up to 59 months did not demonstrate breast cancer in any of the patients with benign cytologic diagnosis after FNAB.

As we screen greater numbers of women with mammography and obtain more data on FNAB, the use of this procedure for nonpalpable lesions may gain greater acceptance. Such a procedure has the potential to reduce the number of surgical biopsies performed. However, the false-negative rates of approximately 9% reported for FNAB of palpable lesions now prohibit widespread use of FNAB for nonpalpable lesions.[14, 15] A positive diagnosis of malignancy in a nonpalpable lesion made preoperatively by FNAB may, however, be of help in planning appropriate therapy, but patients with negative cytologic studies after FNAB continue to need close follow-up or biopsy.

References

1. Moskowitz M: Screening is not diagnosis. Radiology 133:265–268, 1979.
2. Meyer JE, Kopans DB, Stomper PC, et al: Occult breast abnormalities: Percutaneous preoperative needle localization. Radiology 50:335–337, 1984.

3. Frankl G, Rosenfield DD: Breast xeroradiography: An analysis of our first 17 months. Ann Surg 178:676–679, 1973.

4. Price JL, Butler PD: Stereoscopic measurement in mammography. Br J Radiol 44:901, 1971.

5. Horns JW, Arndt RD: Percutaneous spot localization of nonpalpable breast lesions. AJR 127:253–256, 1976.

6. Kopans DB, Meyer JE: Versatile spring hookwire breast lesion localizer. AJR 138:586–587, 1982.

7. Kopans DB, Lindfors KK, McCarthy KA, et al: Spring hookwire breast lesion localizer: Use with rigid-compression mammographic systems. Radiology 157:537–538, 1985.

8. Homer MJ: Nonpalpable breast lesion localization using a curved-end retractable wire. Radiology 157:259–260, 1985.

9. Yagan R, Wiesen E, Bellon EM: Mammographic needle localization of lesions seen in only one view. AJR 144:911–916, 1985.

10. Kopans DB, Meyer JE: Computed tomography guided localization of clinically occult breast carcinoma—the "N" skin guide. Radiology 145:211–212, 1982.

11. Kopans DB, Meyer JE, Lindfors KK, et al: Breast sonography to guide cyst aspiration and wire localization of occult solid lesions. AJR 143:489–492, 1984.

12. Bradbeer JW: Out-patient diagnosis of breast cancer. Br J Surg 72:927–928, 1985.

13. Somers RG, Young GP, Kaplan MJ, et al: Fine-needle aspiration biopsy in the management of solid breast tumors. Arch Surg 120:673–676, 1985.

14. Minkowitz S, Moskowitz R, Khafif RA, et al: Tru-Cut needle biopsy of the breast. An analysis of its specificity and sensitivity. Cancer 57:320–323, 1986.

15. Wollenberg NJ, Caya JG, Clowry, LJ: Fine needle aspiration cytology of the breast. A review of 321 cases with statistical evaluation. Acta Cytol 29:425–429, 1985.

16. Kehler M, Albrechtsson U: Mammographic fine needle biopsy of non-palpable breast lesions. Acta Radiol Diagn 25:273–276, 1984.

Ultrasonographic Aspiration and Biopsy Techniques

John P. McGahan, M.D., and
Fred Hanson, M.D.

Aspiration biopsy techniques performed under radiographic control are not new. In 1939, Blady described his experience with aspiration biopsy techniques in difficult locations using roentgenographic guidance.[1] Interest in aspiration biopsy has increased with the development of newer imaging methods and the refinement of cytologic techniques. Although palpable lesions do not require imaging, ultrasonography and computerized tomography (CT) can visualize solid organs in detail and allow for precise needle placement in nonpalpable deeper lesions. The selection of an imaging modality for needle placement is often dependent on the degree of operator familiarity with a particular procedure. In many situations, however, there are specific advantages of one imaging modality over another in the performance of a biopsy.

Sonographic guidance systems are relatively inexpensive as compared with CT. In general, the cost of sophisticated ultrasonographic systems is approximately one-tenth that of CT. Ultrasonographic equipment therefore is ideal for the outpatient setting and may produce significant cost savings when compared with comparable CT examinations. Furthermore, it can be performed relatively quickly. The time for a complete aspiration biopsy is usually not much longer than for a routine ultrasonographic examination. Because ultrasonographic systems are mobile, aspiration biopsies can be performed anywhere within the outpatient facility.[2]

An important recent technical development is a variety of ultrasonographic needle guidance systems that allow for direct sonographic visualization of the biopsy needle as it passes into a target lesion.[3-5] These newer needle guidance systems may be used with either linear array or sector real-time scanners (Fig. 6–1).[3-5] Newer needles that have been developed are more readily imaged by real-time ultrasonography as they are being placed into a target lesion (Fig. 6–2).[5, 6] The visual control provided by ultrasonography increases the accuracy of needle placement and avoids the inadvertent entrance into vital intervening structures. In addition, changes in the size or shape of a lesion can be monitored by the ultrasonographic biopsy system. A major disadvantage of ultrasonography is its inability to image structures obscured by bone, air, or bowel gas.

TECHNIQUE

Patient Preparation

Proper patient consent must be obtained and the procedure explained in detail, including its risks, benefits, and any alternatives. The patient should be questioned concerning easy bruising, abnormal bleeding during tooth extraction or recent surgery, and any medications that may prolong bleeding time. Coagulation studies including prothrombin time (PT), partial thromboplastin time (PTT), and platelet count, as well as hematocrit, should be routinely obtained. A formalized bleeding time is determined only in patients with a history of bleeding. It should be emphasized that these studies should be obtained at the most recent clinic visit *before* the needle biopsy.

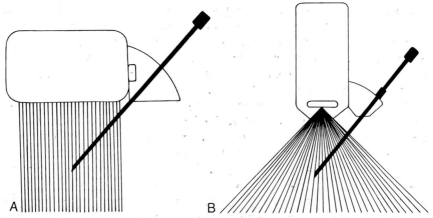

Figure 6–1. Biopsy guide attachment. Biopsy guide attachments that may be used for either linear array *(A)* or sector *(B)* real-time ultrasonography that allow visualization of the needle as it crosses the path of the ultrasound beam. (From McGahan JP [ed]: Controversies in Ultrasound. New York, Churchill Livingstone, 1987, pp 249–267. With permission.)

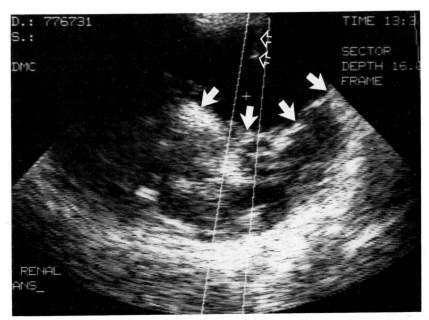

Figure 6–2. Perirenal cyst aspiration. 22-gauge needle (open arrows) between biopsy guide cursors entering right perirenal cyst. Closed arrows outline the wall of the cyst.

Patients usually are asked to fast for at least 6 hours before the examination. Since patients are often uncomfortable, apprehensive, and sometimes in slight pain during the procedure, premedication with a combination of intramuscular meperidine (Demerol) and hydroxyzine hydrochloride (Vistaril) or a small amount of diazepam (Valium) orally may be helpful. An intravenous line is generally unnecessary but should be considered for elderly patients or for any patient with whom a problem is anticipated. The use of analgesia and an intravenous line is determined by the patient, the situation, the possible difficulty, and the site of biopsy.

GUIDANCE SYSTEMS

Ultrasound-guided biopsy can be aided by either of two methods. The first method uses an ultrasonographic probe to select the site of the patient's skin for puncture. The skin is marked with pressure from the hub of the needle, and the angle and depth of the puncture are preselected from the ultrasonographic image. The probe is removed, and the patient is prepared and draped. Real-time or static B-mode ultrasonography can be used. The patient must suspend respiration in the same position in which the ultrasonographic image was obtained. This is extremely important when dealing with lesions close to the hemidiaphragm, where large excursions occur with respiration.

A second method of ultrasonographic localization is the use of a sonographic guidance system allowing direct needle visualization. The patient is prepared and draped after scanning, and a sterile ultrasonographic probe is placed on the skin over the selected area. The transducer is usually not sterilized, but a sterile prefitted glove is placed over the probe (Fig. 6–3). Static B-mode ultrasonography or real-time ultrasonography with a biopsy guide can then be used to guide the needle. A biopsy guide is attached to the transducer, the skin is anesthetized, and the needle is inserted under ultrasonographic guidance into the target lesion

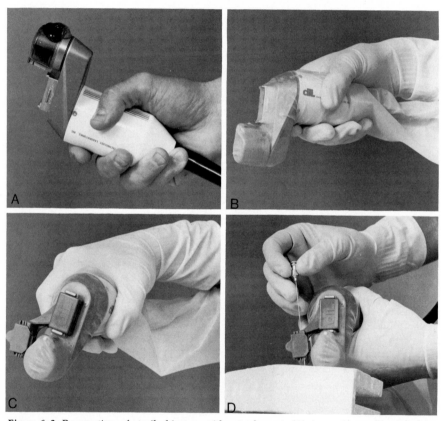

Figure 6–3. Preparation of sterile biopsy guide attachment. *(A)* Acoustic coupling medium (gel) is placed on the head of the ultrasound probe. *(B)* The sterile glove is placed over the ultrasound probe. *(C)* The sterile biopsy guide is attached to the ultrasound probe. *(D)* The needle is inserted through the biopsy guide attachment into the targeted lesion. The needle path is monitored by the biopsy guide cursor as seen on the video screen and demonstrated in Figure 6–2. (From McGahan JP [ed]: Controversies in Ultrasound. New York, Churchill Livingstone, 1987, pp 249–267. With permission.)

(Fig. 6–3). Sterile gel or povidone-iodine solution can be used as an acoustic coupling medium. This method of direct needle guidance allows complete visualization of the needle and is especially useful in biopsy of very small lesions.[5, 6]

Although these needle guidance systems are theoretically ideal for biopsy, pitfalls include a limited needle access route, awkwardness of the guidance systems, needle deflection, and a lack of needle visualization. Needle guides placed laterally to the ultrasonographic probe increase the overall size of the instrumentation. This latter factor may be a minor problem when performing biopsies in areas of limited access, such as between the ribs. In addition, such systems are slightly cumbersome as you must simultaneously hold the probe in one hand for imaging while placing the biopsy needle with the opposite hand. In some situations, this technique may require two individuals to perform the biopsy. Methods for improving needle visualization are discussed in the following paragraphs.

NEEDLE SELECTION

A variety of puncture needles may be used with ultrasonographic guidance. In general, smaller needles produce smaller specimens. The corollary to this guide for needle selection is that, in general, there usually is an increased incidence of complications with larger needles.[7–9] Needle selection may be predetermined by the type of specimen desired. A small-bore (22- or 23-gauge) needle is usually adequate for cytologic diagnosis, whereas a larger-bore needle (14- to 16-gauge) is needed for histologic diagnosis. A 22- or 23-gauge needle may be most appropriate for cytologic diagnosis of liver metastases but may be inadequate for evaluating hepatic architecture to diagnose postnecrotic cirrhosis. If a core of tissue is needed, a larger-bore needle such as a long Menghini (2 mm outside diameter) or a Tru-Cut is used. Thus, the advantage of a larger specimen obtained with a larger-bore needle must be weighed against the associated increase in complications.[8]

A needle with a beveled edge (Chiba, spinal) is more suitable than a nonbeveled needle (Greene) (Fig. 6–4).[7] A small-caliber needle (22- to 23-gauge) can be placed in any hollow viscus (bowel) in the abdomen without causing damage. This is important in pancreatic biopsies, when it is usually necessary to transgress the stomach to obtain pancreatic tissue. However, in order to avoid the risk of contamination and infection of the fluid collection, not even a small-gauge needle should be passed through the bowel into a sterile fluid collection.

Compared to larger, stiffer needles, small-bore needles (22- to 23-gauge) are more easily deflected when passing through subcutaneous

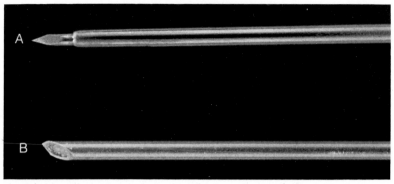

Figure 6–4. Comparison between nonbeveled Greene needle including inner stylet **(A)** and beveled Chiba-type needle **(B)**.

tissue. This problem may be solved by using a larger (18-gauge, 3.8-cm) needle as a guide through the subcutaneous tissue. The smaller-gauge needle may then be placed through the larger-bore needle.

The smaller needles are not easily visualized with real-time biopsy guides, and usually only the tip of a standard 22- or 23-gauge needle is seen. Improvement in the visualization of the needle may be obtained by gently jiggling the needle or moving the inner stylet up and down. If it is thought that the placement of the biopsy needle has deflected out of the plane of the image, then rocking the transducer into the path of the needle may improve visualization. Other less common methods to improve ultrasound needle localization include passage of a small gauge guidewire (0.018 inch) through the 22-gauge needle or injection of saline or air. However, after air is injected through the biopsy needle it tends to act as an acoustic barrier to visualization of deeper structures. Recently introduced roughened Teflon-coated needles have greatly improved ultrasound needle visualization, allowing visualization of the entire needle rather than just the tip (Figs. 6–5, 6–6).

MODIFIED COAXIAL TECHNIQUE

Another technique used with ultrasonic guidance is the modified coaxial needle technique. Under ultrasonographic or CT guidance, a 23-gauge needle is first passed into a suspected lesion. After proper positioning, the inner stylet of the needle is removed. The hub of the needle is either cut with a sterile wire cutter or broken by holding the proximal needle in the left hand and bending the hub back and forth. The 23-gauge needle, with proper depth, acts as a guide for the 19-gauge needle from the Greene biopsy set (Fig. 6–7).[10] A 22-gauge needle with a removable hub and an 18-gauge needle that will pass over the smaller needle can also be

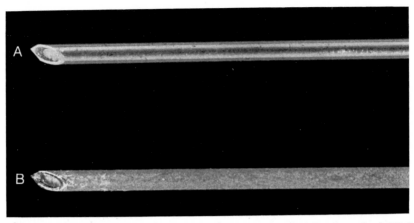

Figure 6–5. Comparison between standard 22-gauge Chiba needle **(A)** and roughened Teflon-coated 22-gauge needle **(B)**.

used.[11] In either system, once the 18- or 19-gauge needle is positioned, multiple passes with a 22- or 23-gauge needle may be made without violating the intervening structures (Fig. 6–7). The 18- or 19-gauge needle may also be used for biopsy to obtain a larger specimen than the smaller needles. Properly used, the modified coaxial technique will incorporate the advantages of the small- and large-bore needles and reduce their disadvantages. This technique may be especially useful in small, poorly accessible lesions, which may require more than one pass to obtain proper needle position.

OTHER NEEDLE TECHNIQUES

Other techniques for biopsy include the fan biopsy technique and use of tandem needles. In the fan biopsy, multiple needles are passed in a fan-type configuration (Fig. 6–8).[12–13] This technique can be used for the biopsy of diffuse liver metastases without a focal nodule. For the tandem needle technique, a second needle is passed parallel to the first needle, which has already been placed into an organ (Fig. 6–9).[14] The modified coaxial technique, the fan technique, and tandem needles may also be used with other guidance systems such as CT.

SPECIMEN HANDLING

When the needle is properly positioned, aspiration is performed by applying 8 to 10 ml of negative suction with a hand-held syringe. Several 1-cm up-and-down movements are simultaneously made within the le-

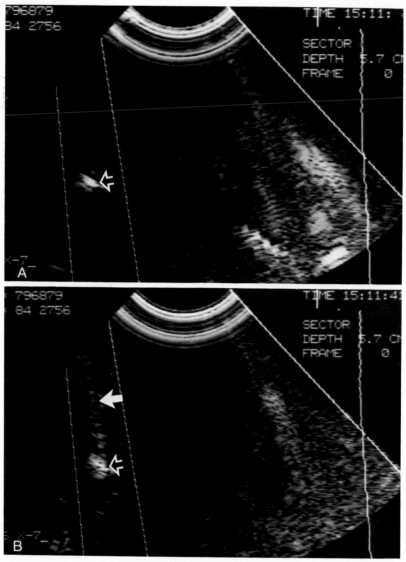

Figure 6–6. Sonographic needle visualization. *(A)* A 22-gauge Chiba needle is passed through the biopsy guide into a beaker of water. This shows only the needle tip (open arrow). *(B)* With similar gain settings, a roughened Teflon-coated 22-gauge needle is passed through the biopsy guide, showing not only the tip of the needle (open arrows) but also the roughened shaft of the needle (arrow). (From McGahan JP [ed]: Controversies in Ultrasound. New York, Churchill Livingstone, 1987, pp 249–267. With permission.)

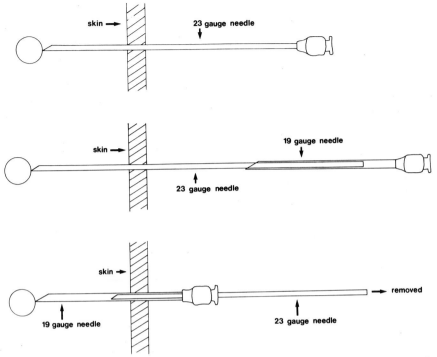

Figure 6–7. Modified coaxial technique. (Top) A 23-gauge needle is passed percutaneously to the edges of a suspected lesion. (Middle) After removing the inner stylet and hub of the 23-gauge needle, a 19-gauge needle may be passed over the 23-gauge needle to the edge of the suspected lesion. (Bottom) The 23-gauge needle is removed, and multiple biopsies may be performed with either a 22- or 23-gauge needle without violating intervening vital structures. (With permission of McGahan JP: Radiology 153:257–258, 1984.)

sion. A rotatory-type motion of the needle may be helpful.[14, 15] This rotatory motion and the use of a larger needle may produce a histologic specimen or core of tissue. Release of the negative suction as the needle is removed from the lesion is necessary so as not to aspirate more proximal contents. Aspirating the tumor sample into the syringe will make it difficult to remove and cause fragmentation, and thus will ruin the cytologic specimen.

To help maintain needle suction and simultaneously provide needle movement, special suction guns have been designed to hold the needle in place and provide negative suction with ample freedom for needle control. There are also some needle-syringe systems that provide needle suction without the operator's simultaneously holding the hub of the syringe and the tip of the needle (Fig. 6–10).

After a specimen is obtained, it is given to a cytologist who is present during the biopsy. The cytologist carefully removes the specimen from

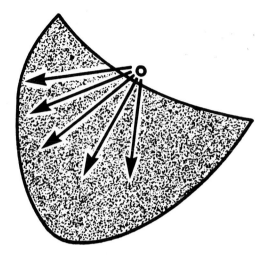

Figure 6–8. Fan needle technique. Multiple needles may be placed from one focus in a fan-type configuration for detection of nondiscrete liver metastases.

Figure 6–9. Tandem needle technique. A second needle is passed parallel with the first needle, which has already been placed into a suspected lesion.

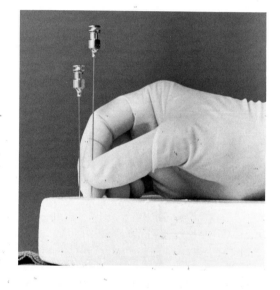

the syringe and smears it on a clear glass slide. A variety of different stains can be used. Wet fixation in alcohol, preparations of filters or cell blocks, and Papanicolaou stains are usually preferred.[16] Air-dried Romanovsky's stained smears from the aspirate can also be used. At our institution, we place on the specimen one drop of toluidine blue in 50% alcohol. This stains and fixes the specimen on the slide for immediate microscopic review. The cytologist views the slide under oil immersion or dry high power at approximately 400× magnification.

At the time of the biopsy, the cytologist checks for adequacy of the specimen and for abnormal cytologic findings. The best specimens are

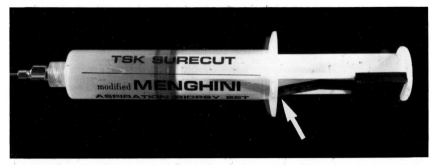

Figure 6–10. TSK Surecut modified Menghini needle with small snap on the inner hub of the syringe, which will allow for needle suction without operator assistance.

obtained when there is little blood to obscure visualization of abnormal cells. The cytologist should inform the radiologist of the adequacy of the specimen and should identify atypical cells, thus allowing termination of biopsy. This reduces the number of passes. If infection is suspected, part of the material is preserved for proper bacteriologic, tubercular, or fungal staining and culture.

SPECIFIC AREAS OF THE BODY

Head and Neck

Lesions of the head and neck are readily accessible to needle aspiration biopsy techniques. Target areas include lesions of the scalp, ear, face, neck, and orbit. The use of ultrasonography is limited in fine-needle aspiration (FNA) of head and neck lesions, as the majority of these lesions are readily palpable. However, ultrasound-guided biopsy of lesions that are not easily palpable or that are in critical (vascular) regions may be successful in obtaining useful cytologic information.

Solbiati and colleagues recently described the use of ultrasonographic biopsy guidance system by FNA to detect parathyroid adenomas.[6] These tumors are usually small (1 cm) and often deep to the thyroid, but they can be clearly visualized with ultrasonography (Fig. 6–11). In Solbiati's series, ultrasound-guided FNA had an accuracy rate of 86.5% in suspected parathyroid adenomas. Techniques for aspiration have been previously described in this chapter.

Thyroid nodules are usually discovered by palpation, so imaging is not needed to aid FNA. When nonpalpable lesions are discovered by radionuclide thyroid scan or ultrasonography, however, needle aspiration can be guided by sonographic techniques. Ultrasonography may help determine the anatomy and multiplicity of lesions.

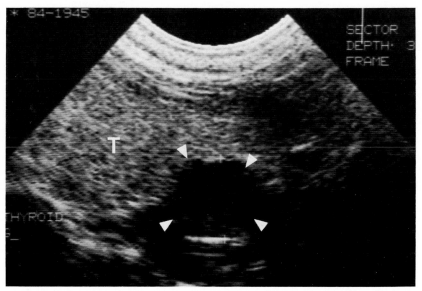

Figure 6–11. Parathyroid adenoma. Longitudinal scan through the inferior pole of the right thyroid **(T)** shows a 1-cm anechoic lesion that corresponds to a small parathyroid adenoma (arrowheads). Fine-needle aspiration may be used in definitive diagnosis of such cases.

Although sensitivity rates for FNA of thyroid neoplasms are 88% and specificity is 80%, there are pitfalls with aspiration of the thyroid.[17, 18] There are a number of neoplasms that are indeterminate as to benignity or malignancy with FNA. A significant number of indeterminate cellular thyroid nodules are actually malignant, with the reported rates of malignancy varying from 18 to 60%.[19-21] In these cases of thyroid nodules indeterminate by FNA, follow-up with thyroid suppression, nodule disappearance or decrease in size by ultrasonography following aspiration, and repeat biopsy with large-bore needles all are important in supporting nonoperative therapy.[18, 19] Other investigators advocate surgery in the indeterminate group.[21]

Ultrasonography has also been helpful for imaging lymphadenopathy, parotid masses, and submandibular gland masses.[22] Although data have been published on aspiration and biopsy of the parotid and other neck masses, only minimal work has been published on ultrasonic guidance in these areas.[23-26] This is because most of the head and neck lesions are easily palpable, requiring no image guidance system.

Chest

Until recently, the sonographic applications of outpatient biopsy procedures of the chest have been limited because the air within the lungs acts as an acoustic barrier. However, ultrasonography may be useful in needle aspiration of diseases of the lung and pleura.[27, 28] Izumi and colleagues described a linear array needle biopsy unit used in the biopsy of chest lesions.[27] Most of the lesions were intrapulmonary tumors, but mediastinal masses were also included. All masses abutted the chest wall, producing a good acoustic window. Biopsy using a 22-gauge needle was performed satisfactorily without complication. Others have shown this technique to have application to other pulmonary lesions abutting the pleura.[28]

Outpatient thoracentesis using ultrasonic guidance may also have broad application. This procedure can easily be done with a 3.8-cm, 22-gauge injection needle with a syringe attached to supply suction. This technique is similar to previously described techniques and consists of marking an area of interest, inserting the needle over a rib with ultrasonic guidance, and aspirating the pleural fluid. Thoracentesis under ultrasonic guidance has been proved to be a quick and safe technique, compared with blind aspiration.[2]

Pleural (ultrasound-guided) biopsies may easily be performed as an outpatient procedure. This is a more invasive procedure than simple fluid aspirations, because of the size and configuration of the cutting needle. The biopsy is best performed in cases in which there is a small amount of pleural fluid. A large-gauge Cope cutting needle is used to obtain a sample by snaring tissue as the needle is removed from the pleura. This specimen is adequate for histologic diagnosis but is associated with a higher complication rate than FNA.[29, 30] To detect a hemo- or pneumothorax, a follow-up chest x-ray is always performed immediately after biopsy and again several hours later.

Breast

Percutaneous breast biopsy is an accurate clinical technique for diagnosing breast malignancy.[31–34] It is also a less expensive method than excisional biopsy.[33] Most percutaneous biopsy or needle localization for excisional biopsy is performed under mammographic guidance. Ultrasonography may help to differentiate between cystic and solid discrete masses.[35] Thin needles may also be used for aspiration of breast cysts. Once breast cysts are localized, aspiration is a safe, simple, and economical procedure. The risk of overlooking an associated carcinoma is low.[31] As ultrasonographic breast-imaging techniques become more refined, this imaging modality will become more important in diagnostic aspiration of diseases of the breast.[36, 37]

Liver

FNA biopsy of the liver is a safe and accurate method for cytologic diagnosis of malignancy. Ultrasound guidance has advantages over blind liver biopsies (Figs. 6–12 and 6–13). Either conventional or FNA liver biopsy can be performed as an outpatient procedure. The biopsy is done in the morning, and the patient is monitored closely for the first few hours, especially after undergoing conventional or large-bore needle biopsy. The patient should be able to resume normal activity before being discharged.[43] If a percutaneous needle biopsy is performed for suspected metastatic liver disease, FNA is safe and has a high diagnostic yield. However, if the liver biopsy is used to diagnose diffuse liver disease (postnecrotic cirrhosis), a histologic specimen is needed. Use of a large-bore needle, such as a 14- to 16-gauge Menghini, Tru-Cut, or Vim-Silverman, is the most reliable means of obtaining larger specimens needed for histologic examination.

Using FNA techniques, the diagnosis of malignant liver disease has shown a sensitivity rate of approximately 80%.[14, 38, 39] More recent studies have shown a higher diagnostic yield with use of 18-gauge needles than with 22-gauge needles in the liver, without significant increase in morbidity or mortality.[8, 9] The modified coaxial technique may be helpful in this respect, incorporating the advantages of a 19- and 22-gauge needle.[10]

Whichever system is used, ultrasonic guidance can significantly increase the diagnostic yield and decrease the complication rate. Greiner

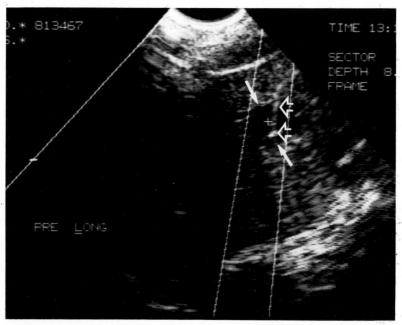

Figure 6–12. Infected biloma. Teflon-coated 22-gauge needle (open arrows) being inserted into 1-cm cystic lesion (between arrows) in the left lobe of the liver, corresponding to an infected biloma.

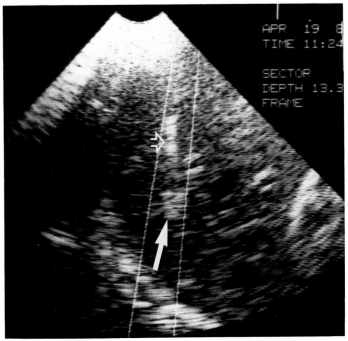

Figure 6–13. Liver hemangioma. Teflon-coated 22-gauge needle (open arrow) being inserted with biopsy guide attachment into 1-cm echogenic lesion in the right lobe of the liver (arrow).

and Franken compared liver biopsy techniques using blind biopsy and ultrasound-guided biopsy with a Menghini needle.[40] Ultrasonographic knowledge of liver topography reduced the complication rate in this series from 1.4 to 0.2% and reduced the need for analgesia from 4.5 to 1.1%. In cases of Chilaiditi's syndrome, the bowel may be interposed between the liver and the abdominal wall, a situation that could be disastrous if a blind biopsy were performed. The use of ultrasonographic needle guidance systems with fine needles has shown an increased accuracy rate of cytologic reading of malignancy, as high as 95% in large series.[41, 42]

Nondiagnostic needle aspiration biopsies are not uncommon, especially when the cytologist is unable to differentiate between a low-grade malignancy and a benign lesion. In these cases, a repeat needle biopsy or use of a larger-bore needle may be helpful. The diagnostic accuracy should improve with use of commercial biopsy systems and roughened Teflon-coated needles.

Using conventional (non-FNA) liver biopsy techniques, Terry reported a series of 10,600 biopsies with a 0.1% mortality rate and 4% morbidity rate.[44] Perrault and colleagues reported significant hypotension after use of a Tru-Cut needle in 3% of cases.[45] Using the Menghini needle in a series of 23,282 and 79,381 patients, the mortality rates were 0.017 and 0.015%, respectively.[46, 47] The overall mortality rate with conventional liver biopsy technique is estimated to be between 0.01 and 0.1%, with a significant morbidity rate of 1 and 4%. In comparison, the complication rate of FNA is approximately one-tenth of this conventional technique.[48]

Hemorrhage is the major potential complication of percutaneous needle liver biopsy. Two delayed hemorrhages (one fatal, 15 days after biopsy) following percutaneous liver biopsy using a 14-gauge needle have been reported.[49] This type of complication would not have been avoided even if the procedure had been performed on an inpatient basis, as the patient would have been discharged before the bleeding occurred. Although hemorrhage may be a problem with the use of larger-bore needles, fine needles have been used safely for the biopsy of such potentially dangerous lesions as cavernous hemangiomas.[50] When performing any needle biopsy of the abdomen, care must be taken to avoid puncture of the inferior epigastric artery, which usually runs along the lateral two-thirds of the rectus sheath. Another potential complication with the use of FNA is biopsy-induced anaphylaxis, which has been reported with the puncture of echinococcal liver cysts. Serologic testing for echinococcus is recommended before puncturing a suspicious liver cyst. A recent series has described not only puncture of such echinococcal cysts but complete drainage with percutaneous technique without complications.[51]

Other potential complications of percutaneous needle aspiration of the liver include pneumothorax, bile peritonitis, peritonitis secondary to bowel puncture, and tumor seeding. These complications may occur with larger needles but are extremely rare with smaller needles. Pain, fever, and mild hemorrhage have been reported when performing FNA of the liver.[48]

Pancreas

Ultrasonographic biopsy of the pancreas can be safely performed as an outpatient procedure. Fine needles must be used in pancreatic biopsy, because the stomach is often transgressed during the anterior approach. Studies of percutaneous cytodiagnosis of abdominal masses by ultrasound-guided FNA biopsy have shown an accuracy rate of 93% in the pancreas as compared with 95% in the liver.[41, 52] The use of fine-needle ultrasonographic guidance systems in pancreatic biopsy has also been shown to have a high diagnostic accuracy (Fig. 6–14).[42]

Complications from fine-needle biopsies of the pancreas are potentially more serious than they are for liver biopsies. One death, secondary to fatal necrotizing pancreatitis, has been reported with FNA of the pancreas.[53] Spread of tumor along the needle tract with pancreatic cancers

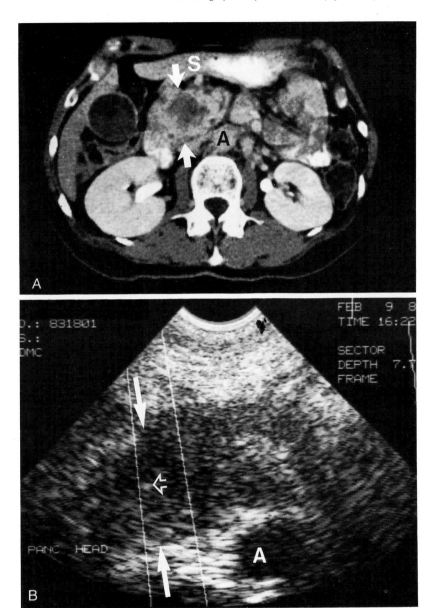

Figure 6–14. Pancreatic carcinoma. CT scan showing large inhomogeneous lesion in the head of the pancreas (between arrows). The lumen of the stomach must be transgressed for this lesion to be biopsied through the anterior abdominal wall. **S,** stomach; **A,** aorta. *(B)* Real-time ultrasonography with biopsy guide using a 22-gauge non–Teflon-coated needle showing just the tip of the needle (open arrow) in the enlarged pancreatic head (between arrows) corresponding to a pancreatic carcinoma. **A,** aorta.

has also been reported.[14, 54] Other potential complications include nonfatal pancreatitis, peritonitis, and hemorrhage.[55] In general, if a lesion is present in the pancreas and in another abdominal area, it might be best to consider biopsy of the other mass before biopsy of the pancreatic lesion.

A recent report described ultrasound-guided percutaneous fine-needle biopsy of the pancreatic duct followed by cholangiography.[56] Using this technique, pancreatic fluid can be aspirated for cytologic diagnosis. This technique is not widely used, and more experience should be gained before considering this a routine procedure.

Gastrointestinal Tract

Ultrasonography has been shown to be useful for visualizing the thickened hollow abdominal viscus in cases of malignancy. Carcinoma of the colon or stomach can be visualized as a thickened wall with a hypoechoic center corresponding to the bowel mucosa. This has been termed the pseudo-kidney sign.[57] Because these lesions are visualized by ultrasonography, percutaneous FNA of such lesions can be performed. Klann and colleagues biopsied 16 cases of gastrointestinal carcinoma verified by operation, with a sensitivity of 94%.[55] Although many of these patients were hospitalized because of their illness, biopsies may be performed on an outpatient basis.

Spleen

There are few reports of FNA of the spleen. In a series of patients with heterogeneous liver scintigraphy (^{99m}Tc-sulfur-colloid) and negative sonograms, Jansson and colleagues performed FNA under sonographic guidance using an 0.8-mm outer diameter (21-gauge) needle without major complications.[58] They used FNA to diagnose spleen infiltration in 2 of 36 Hodgkin's, 9 of 61 non-Hodgkin's, and suspected lymphoma in 2 of the 7 cases in each category. Unfortunately, in the spleen, malignant lymphocytes are often difficult to differentiate from normal lymphocytes. The problem of a small tissue sample in relation to the diagnosis of lymphoma has also been reported by others.[59]

Lymph Nodes

The diagnostic accuracy of retroperitoneal and pelvic lymph node biopsies varies from 65 to 90%.[60] This wide variation is due to the need to obtain a large tissue sample, required to accurately diagnose the cell patterns in lymphoma.[59]

Imaging techniques that can be used to aid biopsy in suspected cases of malignant node enlargement include fluoroscopy after lymphangiography, and CT or ultrasonography. Ultrasonography can be used when adenopathy is sonographically visualized (Fig. 6–15). Biopsy techniques are similar to those previously described. Care must be taken to avoid biopsy of the aorta or inferior vena cava. Real-time ultrasonic needle-guidance systems show these structures to be pulsating.

Renal/Adrenal

Renal biopsies are performed either for cases of suspected malignancy or for histologic diagnosis of renal architecture. Large-bore (Vim-Silverman, Tru-Cut, or Jamshidi) renal biopsy needles can be used for the diagnosis of architectural abnormalities, whereas thin needles are often satisfactory for cytologic diagnosis. Larger-size needles are often needed to diagnose renal malignancy invading or metastatic to the liver, and therefore the modified coaxial technique may be helpful in this region.[10] Whatever needle is used, ultrasonography is helpful in marking the site and depth of the renal cortex. Ultrasonographic needle biopsy guides have also been used to direct renal biopsy. Renal biopsies were at first performed under fluoroscopic guidance.[61] In the 1970s, B-scan ultrasonography was introduced.[62] Ultrasonography is much safer than fluoroscopy for the patient and staff, since it uses no ionizing radiation. It can be used for patients with poor renal function because iodinated contrast material is not used. Ultrasonography may also be useful to demonstrate complications of renal biopsy (Fig. 6–16).

Using B-scan techniques, renal tissue was recovered in 95% of the cases described by Afschrift and colleagues.[63] In another promising report, glomeruli were recovered in all patients undergoing kidney biopsy using a real-time ultrasonographic biopsy guide attachment.[61] The biopsy needle (Tru-Cut) was similar to the needles used in other reports. The complication rate of the 41 patients in this series was extremely low. Only one patient had back pain, and two patients had microscopic hematuria. There were no reported clinical complications, decreased hematocrits, transfusions, postbiopsy hematomas, or cases of hypertension.[61]

Complications of large-bore renal biopsy include severe hemorrhage, arteriovenous fistulas, postbiopsy hypertension, eventual nephrectomy, hematoma formation, hematuria, fever, and abdominal tenderness. Recent reports have shown the complication rate to be reduced by approximately 50% in centers switching from fluoroscopy guidance to B-mode ultrasonic guidance.[64]

FNA biopsy of the kidneys and adrenals for suspected malignancy can be performed as previously described. There are few complications if

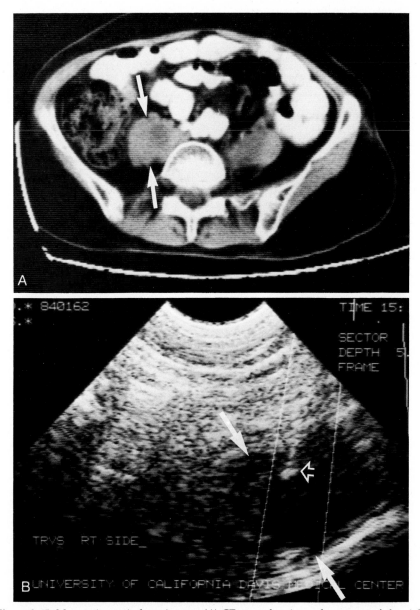

Figure 6–15. Metastatic cervical carcinoma. *(A)* CT scan showing enlargement of the right psoas (between arrows) with associated mild adenopathy. *(B)* Teflon-coated 22-gauge needle (open arrow) being placed into anechoic right psoas (between large arrows), corresponding to metastatic cervical carcinoma. (From McGahan JP [ed]: Controversies in Ultrasound. New York, Churchill Livingstone, 1987, pp 249–267. With permission.)

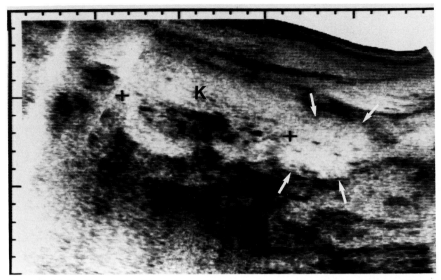

Figure 6–16. Postbiopsy renal hematoma. Prone ultrasonography of the left kidney **(K)** with anechoic area projecting from the inferior pole, which corresponded to postbiopsy hematoma (arrows).

the biopsies are performed with the patient prone. Also, the right adrenal can be biopsied with the needle placed transhepatically.[65] Potential complications of FNA are similar to but less frequent than those described for large-bore needle biopsy of the kidneys. A potential contraindication to biopsy of the adrenal is suspected pheochromocytoma, which can produce a life-threatening blood pressure crisis.[66]

Sonography has long been used for guidance of simple renal cyst puncture.[67] Fluid from the cyst is usually clear and yellow but may become hemorrhagic during a traumatic tap. The protein content of the cyst is quite variable but is usually less than that of plasma. In cases of an infected cyst, the protein level can be very high. There are usually no lipids present in a simple cyst, but their presence is an indicator of malignancy. Lactic dehydrogenase is usually low but has been reported to be elevated in malignancy. Creatinine levels in cysts are usually similar to those of plasma, but the concentrations of urea and glucose tend to be slightly elevated. In cases of suspected malignancy, renal fluid should be cytologically examined. Bacteriologic smears and cultures can be of benefit in cases of possible infection. Injection of air and contrast media into the cyst can be used in combination with plain radiographs. This will help outline the cyst wall and aid in detection of papillary projections within a presumed simple cyst.

Percutaneous nephrostomies are generally inpatient procedures, but readjustments to existing tube systems may be done on an outpatient basis using ultrasonic guidance.[68]

PELVIC DISEASE

There are few descriptions of FNA of the pelvis under ultrasonic guidance. Any pelvic abnormality well visualized with ultrasonography can be aided by sonographic needle guidance (Figs. 6–17 and 6–18). This includes abnormalities of the uterus and ovaries. Aspiration of ovarian masses and other pelvic tumors can usually be performed with minimal discomfort to the patient as an outpatient procedure.[69, 70] The technical problems are similar to those described before, with some problems unique to FNA of ovarian masses. If an ovarian malignancy coexists with a benign cyst, biopsy may sample one area and miss the other. As discussed previously, borderline malignancies are also difficult to evaluate cytologically. This is especially true in cyst aspiration. Laparotomy and careful examination of the ovaries are indicated when the accuracy of sampling is questionable or when there is a strong clinical suspicion of malignancy.

Transrectal sonographic imaging and biopsy of the prostate have been described.[71, 72] Instrumentation has aided in the biopsy of specific nodules within the prostate under ultrasonic guidance.[73, 74]

AMNIOCENTESIS

Diagnostic transabdominal amniocentesis is an accepted and routine outpatient procedure. Use of this procedure has increased dramatically since the mid 1960s because of its demonstrated safety and its aid to geneticists and obstetricians for prenatal genetic studies and the evaluation of fetal well-being and maturity.[75–103]

Historical

Amniocentesis has been used for more than 100 years. Schatz is frequently credited with first using amniocentesis to relieve a case of polyhydramnios; a second report appeared in 1897.[104, 105] It has subsequently been used for determining Rh incompatibility, amniography, prenatal diagnosis, and the evaluation of fetal lung maturity.[106–108]

In 1949, Barr and Bertram reported that morphologic differences in the nuclei of nerve cells of cats could be used to identify the sex of the animal.[109] This report was followed in the mid-1950s by studies by Fuchs and Riis and others, who used amniotic fluid collected at term or at

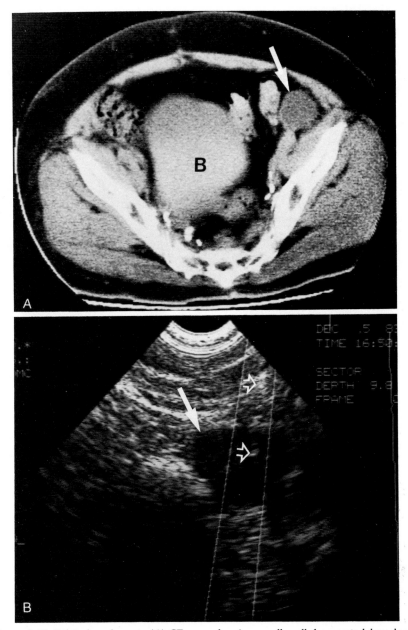

Figure 6–17. Pelvic lymphocyst. *(A)* CT scan showing small well-demarcated low-density area along the high left pelvic sidewall (arrow). **B,** bladder. *(B)* The 22-gauge Teflon-coated needle (open arrows) being inserted into the left-sided anechoic pelvic lesion (arrow), which corresponded to a lymphocyst.

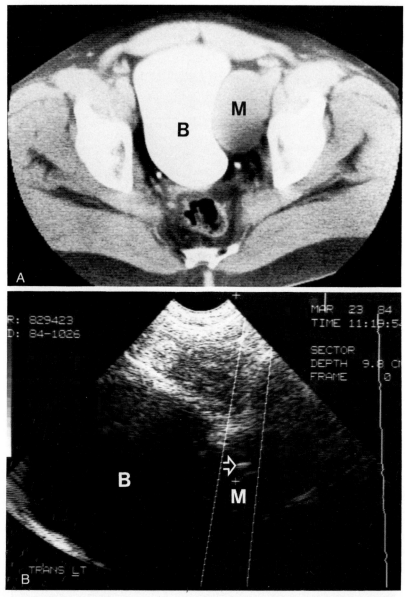

Figure 6–18. Pelvic lymphoma. *(A)* CT scan through the pelvis, demonstrating bladder **(B)** being compressed by a left pelvic mass **(M)**. *(B)* A 23-gauge needle with only a tip visualized (arrow) within the left-sided pelvic mass **(M)**, which corresponded to a lymphoma. **B,** bladder. The modified coaxial technique was used in this case to obtain a larger tissue specimen.[10]

hysterotomy for prenatal sex determination in humans.[110-113] Following these reports, Steele and Breg first successfully determined the viability of human amniotic cells and their culture.[114] Two years later, the first reports of chromosomal and inborn metabolic errors appeared when Jacobsen and Barter demonstrated a 14/15 D/D translocation.[115] In 1968, Valenti and colleagues reported the first trisomy 21 fetus, and Nadler and Dancis reported the first intrauterine diagnosis of galactosemia, muco-polysaccharidosis, and hypervalinemia.[116-118]

Indications

Most midtrimester amniocenteses are performed for genetic indications (Table 6–1). The majority of these procedures are carried out because of maternal age. The need for amniocentesis will increase because of the recent availability of reliable methods for screening large obstetric populations for elevated maternal serum alpha-fetoprotein. Sophisticated centers in several states such as California are instituting large mass prenatal screening programs.[120, 121] Other midtrimester indications for amniocentesis have primarily involved pregnancy termination by injection of hypertonic solutions such as saline and urea or the instillation of intraamniotic prostaglandin $F_2\alpha$.

Diagnostic amniocentesis is also performed in the third trimester of pregnancy (Table 6–2) for cases of Rh factor sensitization and to determine fetal lung maturity in cases of premature labor, premature rupture of the membranes, and repeat elective cesarean section. The mature fetal lung contains surface-active agents that reduce alveolar surface tension and thus confer alveolar stability during deflation. These agents have been identified as phospholipids in the classic work by Gluck and others.[122-124] A fetal lung profile, consisting of a foam stability index (FSI), leci-thin/sphingomyelin ratio (L/S ratio), and the presence of phosphatidyl-glycerol (PG), is performed on the amniotic fluid obtained at amniocentesis.[125] In cases of premature labor and premature rupture of the

Table 6–1
GENETIC INDICATIONS FOR AMNIOCENTESIS

Maternal age 35 or greater
History of a prior child with a chromosomal abnormality
Parent(s) with chromosomal abnormality
Parental carrier state for a metabolic disorder
Maternal carrier of X-linked disorder
Parental carrier state for hemoglobinopathies
History of prior child with neural tube defect
Elevated maternal serum alpha-fetoprotein (AFP)

Table 6–2
OTHER INDICATIONS FOR AMNIOCENTESIS

Rh sensitization
Amniography
Evaluate fetal lung maturity; premature labor
Premature rupture of membranes
Elective cesarean section
Suspected amnionitis
Therapeutic abortion
Polyhydramnios

membranes, amniotic fluid is also sent for Gram stain and bacterial culture to determine the possible cause of the problem and to help determine the subsequent course of patient management.

Genetic studies are occasionally indicated as an aid to obstetric management when significant fetal structural abnormalities are discovered later in pregnancy (such as cystic hygroma, omphalocele, diaphragmatic hernia, osteochondrodysplasia). Polyhydramnios is frequently accompanied by genetic and fetal structural abnormalities. Amniocentesis has been used in attempts to relieve polyhydramnios.[104, 105] Genetic studies are indicated in such situations. Finally, amniocentesis has been used for amniography to outline soft tissue structures such as the placenta, small fetal parts, and the fetal gastrointestinal tract.[108] Other substances in amniotic fluid that have been measured include creatinine, osmolality, δOD 450 (bilirubin), acetylcholinesterase, and the percentage of cells stained orange by Nile blue sulfate to assess fetal maturity.

Technical Aspects of Amniocentesis

Amniocentesis for midtrimester genetic purposes is best done at approximately 16 weeks gestation (since last menstrual period). At this time, the amniotic fluid volume is approximately 200 ml, the uterus is readily accessible above the symphysis pubis, and the peak numbers of viable fetal cells are present in the amniotic fluid.[126–127] Alpha-fetoprotein is best measured between the 15th and 16th weeks. There is ample time for completion of cytogenic studies, thus ensuring that the legal requirements for midtrimester pregnancy termination might be met.

Initially, the patient is counseled by a geneticist or trained genetic counselor who reviews the indications, obtains a genetic history, and explains the procedure of amniocentesis including maternal and fetal risks. They also attempt to allay anxieties and answer all the patient's questions.

Ultrasonography is a vital part of the amniocentesis. At our institution, we employ continuous real-time scanning to monitor needle insertion. The information sought from ultrasonography is listed in Table 6–3 and includes the following: fetal age (biparietal diameter, femur length, abdominal girth, crown-rump measurement); placental localization; multiple gestation; umbilical cord insertion and localization; fetal abnormalities (e.g., neural tube defects, limb abnormalities, omphalocele); uterine fibroids; uterine contractions; amniotic fluid volume (oligohydramnios, polyhydramnios) (Fig. 6–19); fetal heart rate both before and after amniocentesis; needle depth and allowable direction of needle movement if fluid is not readily obtained; and fetal movement patterns. Ultrasonography does not appear to reduce the incidence of bloody taps or the frequency of needle insertions.[93, 131, 132]

Sterile technique is used after ultrasonic localization of the optimal site for amniocentesis. The skin is prepared with povidone-iodine (Betadine)* solution and sterilely draped. A 1% lidocaine HCl (Xylocaine) solution is used for local anesthesia (optional). A 20- or 21-gauge spinal needle is inserted into the amniotic fluid pocket, and 20 to 30 ml of fluid is removed. The first 1 to 2 ml of amniotic fluid is discarded to avoid maternal cell contamination and to clear the needle of any blood encountered in passage through the uterine wall or placenta if it is anterior and unavoidable. Fetal movement and heart rate are carefully recorded after amniocentesis. Three hundred micrograms of Rh immunoglobulin (RhoGAM) is administered to all Rh-negative women unless their partners are Rh negative.[75, 128–130, 133]

The amniotic fluid is transferred to sterile plastic tubes and transported at room temperature to the cytogenetics laboratory. At the time of amniocentesis, ultrasonography is used to avoid transplacental amniocen-

---

*The Purdue Frederick Company: 50 Washington Street, Norwalk, Connecticut 06856

Table 6–3
ULTRASONOGRAPHIC INFORMATION

Fetal age
Placental localization
Multiple gestation
Umbilical cord insertion and location
Fetal location
Fetal abnormalities
Uterine fibroids
Uterine contractions
Amniotic fluid volume (oligo- or polyhydramnios)
Fetal heart rate (before and after TAP)
Bladder localization
Amniotic fluid pocket localization for amniocentesis
Allowable needle depth and movement
Fetal movement patterns

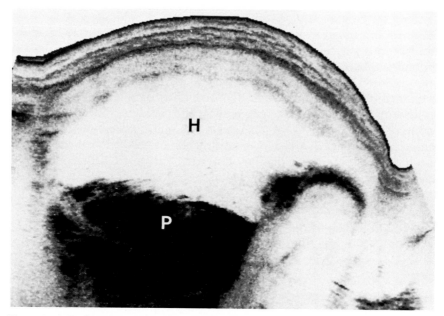

Figure 6–19. Hydramnios. Increased amounts of amniotic fluid **(H)** are noted in this infant with an open neural tube defect. **P,** placenta.

tesis. Anterior placentas have been reported in up to 50% of patients. If the placenta is unavoidable, amniocentesis should be done at a site distant from the umbilical cord insertion. Porreco and colleagues reported a twofold increase in fetal loss with anterior placentation.[82] That has not been the experience at our institution.[134]

Risks of Amniocentesis

The risks of midtrimester amniocentesis have been extensively evaluated.[75–102, 119, 129] Risks can be divided into maternal and fetal categories. It is generally acknowledged that maternal morbidity and mortality are negligible and consist primarily of amniotic fluid leakage, amnionitis, vaginal bleeding, and spontaneous abortion. Fetal injury can be direct, with immediate fetal loss or injury, or indirect, ultimately resulting in fetal wastage. O'Brien recently reviewed published amniocentesis reports from nine representative centers.[95] He concluded that there is a definite fetal risk. He noted increased spontaneous abortion (0.6%), increased neonatal death rate (0.6%), increased total perinatal loss (1.4%), increased antepartum hemorrhage (0.4%), and increased cesarean sections (2.2%). Earlier British reports of increased neonatal respiratory distress and orthopedic problems have not been confirmed.[99]

Future Development

The use of midtrimester genetic amniocentesis is still low. As physicians and the public become aware of the availability of amniocentesis, its use will increase. Personal bias and the small but real risk of complications will, however, prevent routine use.

Chorionic villus biopsy (a transcervical sampling of chorionic villi using a flexible catheter under ultrasonic guidance) is now helping in the first trimester diagnosis of many inherited disorders.[135–137] The procedure is done between the 6th and 8th menstrual weeks, and results are returned within 1 to 3 weeks. Indications for the procedure are identical to midtrimester amniocentesis except for neural tube defects. Risks of fetal loss are unknown but have been reported to be between 5 and 12%, depending on the experience of the center performing the procedure. The risk of other complications is unknown. It appears that the major advantage of chorionic villus biopsy is the ability to diagnose many genetic disorders earlier than amniocentesis (allowing earlier pregnancy termination if needed). The major disadvantages of this procedure appear to be the reduced ability of ultrasonography to detect many unanticipated fetal structural abnormalities at this state of gestation, the inability to diagnose neural tube defects, and the failure to obtain separate genetic material in cases of multiple gestation.

Summary

Midtrimester amniocentesis is a relatively safe outpatient procedure. Maternal morbidity is negligible, accuracy is high, and fetal loss is relatively low. Competent genetic counseling, high-level ultrasonography, and a physician skilled in amniocentesis will result in a fetal loss rate of approximately 0.5%.

ACKNOWLEDGEMENT

Special thanks to Karen Anderson for preparation of this manuscript.

References

1. Blady JV: Aspiration biopsy of tumors in obscure or difficult locations under roentgenoscopic guidance. AJR Rad Ther 42:515–524, 1939.
2. McGahan JP: Aspiration and drainage procedures in the intensive care unit: Percutaneous sonographic guidance. Radiology 154:531–532, 1985.
3. Buonocore E, Skipper GJ: Steerable real-time sonographically guided needle biopsy. AJR 136:387–392, 1981.

4. Holm HH, Als O, Gammelgaard J: Percutaneous aspiration biopsy procedures under ultrasound visualization. *In* Taylor KJW (ed): Clinics in Diagnostic Ultrasound. Vol I. Diagnostic Ultrasound in Gastrointestinal Disease. Churchill Livingstone, New York, 1978, pp 137–149.

5. Otto R, Deyhle P: Guided puncture under real-time sonographic control. Radiology 134:784–785, 1980.

6. Solbiati L, Montali G, Croce F, et al: Parathyroid tumors detected by fine-needle aspiration biopsy under ultrasonic guidance. Radiology 148:793–797, 1983.

7. Andriole JG, Haaga JR, Adams RB, et al: Biopsy needle characteristics assessed in the laboratory. Radiology 148:659–662, 1983.

8. Haaga JR, LiPuma JP, Bryan PJ, et al: Clinical comparison of small- and large- caliber cutting needles for biopsy. Radiology 146:665–667, 1983.

9. Pagani JJ: Biopsy of focal hepatic lesions. Radiology 147:673–675, 1983.

10. McGahan JP: Percutaneous biopsy and drainage procedures in the abdomen using a modified coaxial technique. Radiology 153:257–258, 1984.

11. vanSonnenberg E, Wittich GR, Stauffer AE, et al: Modified coaxial technique to simplify nephrostomy, biliary drainage and biopsies. Presented at the 70th Scientific Assembly and Annual Meeting. Radiol Soc North Am, November 25–30, 1984.

12. Ferrucci JT Jr, Wittenberg J: CT biopsy of abdominal tumors: Aid for lesion localization. Radiology 129:739–744, 1978.

13. Wittenberg J, Mueller PR, vanSonnenberg E, et al: Percutaneous tumor biopsy. *In* Ferrucci JT Jr, Wittenberg J (eds): Interventional Radiology of the Abdomen. Williams & Wilkins, Baltimore, 1981, pp 111–155.

14. Ferrucci JT Jr, Wittenberg J, Mueller PR, et al: Diagnosis of abdominal malignancy by radiologic fine-needle aspiration biopsy. AJR 134:323–330, 1980.

15. Wittenberg J, Mueller PR, Ferrucci JT Jr, et al: Percutaneous core biopsy of abdominal tumor using 22-gauge needles: Further observations. AJR 139:75–80, 1982.

16. Frable WJ: Fine-needle aspiration biopsy: A review. Hum Pathol 14:9–28, 1983.

17. Linsk JA, Franzen S: Head and neck. *In* Linsk JA, Franzen S (eds): Clinical Aspiration Cytology. JB Lippincott, Philadelphia, 1983, pp 41–60.

18. Prinz RA, O'Morchoe PJ, Barbato AL, et al.: Fine-needle aspiration biopsy of thyroid nodules. Ann Surg 198:70–73, 1983.

19. Block MA, Dailey GE, Robb JA: Thyroid nodules indeterminate by needle biopsy. Am J Surg 146:72–78, 1983.

20. Burrow GN: Aspiration needle biopsy of the thyroid. Ann Intern Med 94:536–537, 1981.

21. Belanger R, Guillet F, Matte R, et al: The thyroid nodule: Evaluation of fine-needle biopsy. J Otolaryngol 12:109–111, 1983.

22. Wittich GR, Scheible WF, Hajek PC: Ultrasonography of the salivary glands. Radiol Clin North Am 23:29–37, 1985.

23. Bono A, Chiesa F, Sala L, et al: Fine-needle aspiration biopsy in parotid masses. Tumori 69:417–421, 1983.

24. Gatenby RA, Mulhern CB Jr, Strawitz J: CT-guided percutaneous biopsies of head and neck masses. Radiology 146:717–719, 1983.

25. Sismanis A, Merriam JM, Kline TS, et al: Diagnosis of salivary gland tumors by fine-needle aspiration biopsy. Head Neck Surg 3:482–489, 1981.

26. Young JEM, Archibald SD, Shier KJ: Needle aspiration cytologic biopsy in head and neck masses. Am J Surg 142:484–489, 1981.

27. Izumi S, Tamaki S, Natori H, et al: Ultrasonically guided aspiration needle biopsy in disease of the chest. Am Rev Respir Dis 125:460–464, 1982.

28. Schwerk WB, Dombrowski H, Kalbfleisch H: Ultrasound tomography and sonographically guided needle biopsy of intrathoracic masses. Ultraschall Med 3:212–218, 1982.

29. Cope C, Bernhardt, H: Hook-needle biopsy of pleura, pericardium, peritoneum and synovium. Am J Med 35:189, 1963.

30. Scerbo J, Ketty H, Stone DJ: A prospective study of pleural biopsies. JAMA 218:377, 1971.
31. Dohrmann PJ, Hughes ESR, McDermott FT, et al: Aspiration of breast cysts. Aust NZ J Surg 52:605–607, 1982.
32. Humeniuk V, Kirkpatrick AE, Anderson TJ, et al: Breast localization biopsy. Aust NZ J Surg 52:607–609, 1982.
33. Macksood MJ: Mammography and biopsy of nonpalpable breast lesions: A review of 71 lesions. J Am Osteopath Assoc 83:432–434, 1984.
34. Zagoren AAJ, Waters DJ, Silverman D, et al: Aspiration biopsy for cytologic study of breast masses: An overview. J Am Osteopath Assoc 82:119–123, 1982.
35. McSweeney MB, Murphy CH: Whole breast sonography. Radiol Clin North Am 23:157–167, 1985.
36. McSweeney MB: Sonographic detection of lobular carcinoma. Presented at the 70th Scientific Assembly and Annual Meeting. Radiol Soc North Am, November 25–30, 1984.
37. Merritt CRB, Dempsey PJ: Evaluation and comparison of alternative forms of breast imaging. Presented at the 70th Scientific Assembly and Annual Meeting. Radiol Soc North Am, November 25–30, 1984.
38. Lundquist A: Fine-needle aspiration biopsy for cytodiagnosis of malignant tumor in the liver. Acta Med Scand 188:471–474, 1970.
39. Zornoza J, Wallace S, Ordonez N, et al: Fine-needle aspiration biopsy of the liver. AJR 134:331–334, 1980.
40. Griener L, Franken FH: Die Sonographisch assistierte leberbiopsie—ablosung der bliden leberpunktion: Dtsch Med Wochenschr 108:368–372, 1983.
41. Schwerk WB, Durr HK, Schmitz-Moormann P: Ultrasound guided fine-needle biopsies in pancreatic and hepatic neoplasm. Gastroint Radiol 8:219–225, 1983.
42. Grant EG, Richardson JD, Smirniotopoulos JG, et al: Fine-needle biopsy directed by real-time sonography: Technique and accuracy. AJR 141:29–32, 1983.
43. Shadcherh A: Percutaneous liver biopsy. J Kans Med Soc 82:287–288, 1981.
44. Terry R: Risks of needle biopsy of liver. Br Med J 1:1102–1105, 1972.
45. Perrault J, McGill DB, Ott BJ, et al: Liver biopsy: Complications in 1000 inpatients and outpatients. Gastroenterology 74:103–106, 1978.
46. Thaler H: Uber vorteil and risiko der leberbiopsie methode nach Menghini. Wien Klin Wochenschr 29:533, 1964.
47. Linder H: Grenzen und gefahren der perkutanen leberbiopsie mit der Menghini nadel: erfahrunsen bei 80,000 leberbiopsien. Dtsch Med Wochenschr 92:1751, 1967.
48. Gray WC: A comparison of conventional needle and fine-needle aspiration liver biopsies. J Ind State Med Assoc 76:453–454, 1983.
49. Reichert CM, Weisenthal LM, Klein HG: Delayed hemorrhage after percutaneous liver biopsy. J Clin Gastroenterol 5:263–266, 1983.
50. Livraghi T, Damascelli B, Lombardi C, et al: Risk in fine-needle abdominal biopsy. J Clin Ultrasound 11:77–81, 1983.
51. Bret PM, Bretagnolle M, Fond A, et al: Percutaneous drainage of abscesses and bile ducts in hepatic alveolar echinococcosis (Abstract). Radiol Soc North Am (Chicago), November 13–18, 1983.
52. Porter B, Karp W, Forsberg L: Percutaneous cytodiagnosis of abdominal masses by ultrasound guided fine-needle aspiration biopsy. Acta Radiol [Diagn] 22:663–667, 1981.
53. Evans WK, Ho C-S, McLoughlin MJ, et al: Fatal necrotizing pancreatitis following fine-needle aspiration biopsy of the pancreas. Radiology 141:61–62, 1981.
54. Smith FP, MacDonald JS, Schein S, et al: Cutaneous seeding of pancreatic cancer by skinny needle aspiration biopsy. Arch Intern Med 140:855, 1980.
55. Klann H, Waldthaler A, Voeth C, et al: Perkutane, ultraschallgezielte feinnadelpunkti-

onen (leber, pankreas und darm) und ultraschallgezielte pankreasgangpunktionen. Dtsch Med Wochenschr 108:1503–1507, 1983.

56. Ohto M, Karasawa E, Tsuchiya Y, et al: Ultrasonically guided percutaneous contrast medium injection and aspiration biopsy using a real-time puncture transducer. Radiology 136:171–176, 1980.

57. Yeh HC, Rabinowitz JG: Ultrasonography of gastrointestinal tract. Semin Ultrasound 3:331–347, 1982.

58. Jansson SE, Bondestam S, Heinonen E, et al: Value of liver and spleen aspiration biopsy in malignant diseases when these organs show no signs of involvement in sonography. Acta Med Scand 213:279–281, 1983.

59. Zornoza J, Cabanillas J, Altoff TM, et al: Percutaneous needle biopsy in abdominal lymphoma. AJR 136:97–103, 1981.

60. Bernardino ME: Percutaneous biopsy. AJR 142:41–45, 1984.

61. Backman U, Lindgren PG: Percutaneous renal biopsy with real-time ultrasonography. Scand J Nephrol 16:65–67, 1982.

62. Kristensen JK, Bartels E, Jorgensen HE: Percutaneous renal biopsy under the guidance of ultrasound. Scand J Urol Nephrol 8:223–226, 1974.

63. Afschrift M, Mets T, Matthijs E, et al: A 2-year experience with percutaneous renal biopsy under ultrasonic guidance. Acta Clin Belg 36:237–240, 1981.

64. Altebarmakian VK, Guthinger WP, Yakub YN, et al: Percutaneous kidney biopsies: Complications and their management. Urology 18:118–122, 1981.

65. Price RB, Bernardino ME, Berkman WA, et al: Biopsy of the right adrenal gland by the transhepatic approach. Radiology 148:566, 1983.

66. Lutz H: Ultrasonically-guided fine-needle puncture in gastroenterology. Endoscopy 15:180–182, 1983.

67. Kristensen JK, Jacobsen, GK: Ultrasonically guided puncture of renal mass lesions. *In* Holm HS, Kristensen JK (eds): Ultrasonically Guided Puncture Technique. WB Saunders, Philadelphia, 1980, pp 43–48.

68. Zegel HG, Pollack HM, Banner MP, et al: Percutaneous nephrostomy: Comparison of sonographic and fluoroscopic guidance. AJR 137:925–927, 1981.

69. Ramzy I, Martinez SC, Schantz HD: Ovarian cysts and masses: Diagnosis using fine-needle aspiration. Cancer Detect Prev 4:493–502, 1981.

70. Choo YC, Hsu C, Choy TK, et al: Fine-needle aspiration in gynaecologic oncology. Aust NZ J Obstet Gynaecol 22:226–230, 1982.

71. Maier U, Czerwenka K, Neuhold N: The accuracy of transrectal aspiration biopsy of the prostate: An analysis of 452 cases. Prostate 5:147–151, 1984.

72. Nesi MH, Malloy TR, Carpiniello VL, et al: A comparison of morbidity following transrectal and transperineal prostatic needle biopsy. Surg Gynecol Obstet 156:464–466, 1983.

73. Fornage BD, Touche DH, Deglaire M, et al: Real-time ultrasound-guided prostatic biopsy using a new transrectal linear-array probe. Radiology 146:547–548, 1983.

74. Rifkin MD, Kurtz AB, Goldberg BB: Sonographically guided transperineal prostatic biopsy: Preliminary experience with a longitudinal linear-array transducer. AJR 140:745, 1983.

75. National Institute of Child Health and Human Development: Antenatal diagnosis. Report of a consensus conference. NIH Publication No. 79–1973, 1979.

76. NICHD: The safety and accuracy of midtrimester amniocentesis. NIH Publication No. 78–190, 1978.

77. NICHD National Registry for Amniocentesis Study Group: Midtrimester amniocentesis for prenatal diagnosis: Safety and accuracy. JAMA 236:1471–1476, 1976.

78. Manganiello PD, Byrd JR, Tho PT, et al: A report of the safety and accuracy of midtrimester amniocentesis at the Medical College of Georgia: Eight and one half years' experience. Am J Obstet Gynecol 134:911–916, 1979.

79. Milunsky A, Atkins L: Prenatal diagnosis of genetic disorders. An analysis of experience with 600 cases. JAMA 230:232–235, 1976.

80. Milunsky A: Risk of amniocentesis for prenatal diagnosis. N Engl J Med 293:932–933, 1975.

81. Simpson NE, Dallaire L, Miller JR, et al: Prenatal diagnosis of genetic disease in Canada: Report of a collaborative study. Can Med Assoc J 115:739–746, 1976.

82. Porreco RP, Young PE, Resnik R, et al: Reproductive outcome following amniocentesis for genetic indications. Am J Obstet Gynecol 143:653–660, 1982.

83. Crandall BF, Howard J, Lebherz TB, et al: Followup of 2000 second-trimester amniocenteses. Obstet Gynecol 56:625–628, 1980.

84. Bartsch FK, Lundberg J, Wahlstrom J: One thousand consecutive midtrimester amniocenteses. Obstet Gynecol 55:305–308, 1980.

85. Aula P, Karjalainen O, Teramo K, et al: Safety and accuracy of midtrimester amniocentesis for prenatal diagnosis of genetic disorders. Ann Clin Res 11:156–163, 1979.

86. Wilson MG, Gilman JA, Kellogg B: Prenatal diagnosis by amniocentesis in 800 pregnancies. West J Med 131:201–204, 1979.

87. Golbus MS, Loughman WD, Epstein CJ: Prenatal genetic diagnosis in 3000 amniocenteses. N Engl J Med 300:157–163, 1979.

88. Hsu LYF, Jaffe S, Yahr F, et al: Prenatal cytogenetic diagnosis, first 1000 successful cases. Am J Med Genet 2:365–383, 1978.

89. Galjaard H: European experience with prenatal diagnosis of congenital disease, a survey of 6121 cases. Cytogenet Cell Genet 16:453–467, 1976.

90. Philip J, Bang J: Outcome of pregnancy after amniocentesis for chromosome analysis. Br Med J 2:1183–1184, 1978.

91. Henry GP, Peakman DC, Robinson A: Prenatal genetic diagnosis: Nine years' experience. Obstet Gynecol Surv 33:569–577, 1978.

92. Goldman B, Mashiah S, Serr DM, et al: A survey of amniocentesis in 925 patients at high risk of fetal genetic disorder. Br J Obstet Gynaecol 84:808–814, 1977.

93. Young PE, Matson MR, Jones OW: Amniocentesis for antenatal diagnosis. Review of problems and outcomes in a large series. Am J Obstet Gynecol 125:495–501, 1976.

94. Crandall BF, Lebherz TB: Prenatal genetic diagnosis in 350 amniocenteses. Obstet Gynecol 48:158–162, 1976.

95. O'Brien WF: Midtrimester genetic amniocentesis: A review of the fetal risks. J Reprod Med 29:59–63, 1984.

96. Alexander D, Lowe CU, Seigel D, et al: Risks of amniocentesis. Lancet 2:577–578, 1979.

97. Milunsky A: Hazards of amniocentesis. Lancet 1:546–547, 1979.

98. Park JI, Heller RH, Kaiser RM, et al: Spontaneous abortion after midtrimester amniocentesis. Obstet Gynecol 53:190–194, 1979.

99. Medical Research Council Working Party on Amniocentesis: An assessment of the hazards of amniocentesis. Br J Obstet Gynecol (Suppl 2)85:1–41, 1978.

100. Golbus MS, Conte FA, Schneider EL, et al: Intrauterine diagnosis of genetic defects: Results, problems, and follow-up of one hundred cases in a prenatal genetic detection center. Am J Obstet Gynecol 118:897–905, 1974.

101. Verjaal M, Leschot NJ, Treffers PE: Risk of amniocentesis and laboratory findings in a series of 1500 prenatal diagnoses. Prenat Diag 1:173–181, 1981.

102. Epstein CJ, Golbus MS. Prenatal diagnosis of genetic diseases. Am Sci 65:703–711, 1977.

103. Nadler HL, Gerbie AB: Role of amniocentesis in the intrauterine detection of genetic disorders. N Engl J Med 282:596–599, 1970.

104. Schatz F: Eine besondere art von einseitiger polyhdromnie mit anderseitiger oligohydramnie bei einagueu zwillingen. Arch Gynecol 19:329, 1882.

105. Prochownick L: Beitrage, gur leptre von fruchtivasser und seiner entsehung. Arch Gynecol 11:304, 1897.

106. Bevis DCA: Composition of liquor amnii in haemolytic disease of the newborn. Lancet 2:443, 1950.

107. Bevis DCA: The antenatal prediction of haemolytic disease of the newborn. Lancet 1:395–398, 1952.

108. Menees TO, Miller JD, Holly LE: Amniography: A preliminary report. AJR 24:363–366, 1930.

109. Barr ML, Bertram EG: A morphological distinction between neurones of the male and female and the behavior of the nucleolar satellite during accelerated nucleoprotein synthesis. Nature 163:676–677, 1949.

110. Fuchs F, Riis P: Antenatal sex determination. Nature 177:330, 1956.

111. Makowski EL, Prem KA, Kaiser IH: Detection of sex of fetuses by the incidence of sex chromatin body in nuclei of cells in amniotic fluid. Science 123:542–543, 1956.

112. James F: Sexing foetuses by examination of amniotic fluid. Lancet 1:202–203, 1956.

113. Serr DM, Sachs L, Danon M: Diagnosis of sex before birth using cells from the amniotic fluid. Bull Res Counc Isr 58:137, 1955.

114. Steele MW, Breg WR Jr: Chromosome analysis of human amniotic fluid cells. Lancet 1:383–385, 1966.

115. Jacobsen CB, Barter RH: Intrauterine diagnosis and management of genetic defects. Am J Obstet Gynecol 99:796–807, 1967.

116. Valenti C, Schutta EJ, Kehaty T: Prenatal diagnosis of Down's syndrome. Lancet 2:220, 1968.

117. Nadler HL: Antenatal detection of hereditary disorders. Pediatrics 42:912–918, 1968.

118. Dancis J: The antepartum diagnosis of genetic diseases. J Pediatr 72:301–302, 1968.

119. Read AP, Donnai D, Harris R, et al: Comparison of pregnancy outcome after amniocentesis for previous neural tube defect or raised maternal serum alpha fetoprotein. Br J Obstet Gynaecol 87:372–376, 1980.

120. Macri JN: Alpha fetoprotein prenatal screening in the United States. *In* JE Hadon, JN Macri (eds): Proceedings of Second Scarborough Conference: Alpha Fetoprotein Serum Screening in Pregnancy. Foundation for Blood Research, Scarborough, Maine, 1978.

121. UK Collaborative Study: Maternal serum alpha fetoprotein measurement in antenatal screening for anencephaly and spina bifida in early pregnancy. Lancet 1:1323, 1977.

122. Gluck L, Kulovich MV, Borer RC, et al: Diagnosis of respiratory distress syndrome by amniocentesis. Am J Obstet Gynecol 109:440, 1971.

123. Gluck L, Kulovich MV: Lecithin/sphingomyelin ratios in amniotic fluid in normal and abnormal pregnancy. Am J Obstet Gynecol 115:539, 1973.

124. Gluck L, Kulovich MV, Borer RC, et al: The interpretation and significance of the lecithin/sphingomyelin ratio in amniotic fluid. Am J Obstet Gynecol 120:143, 1974.

125. Cher B, Statland BE, Freer DE: Clinical evaluation of the qualitative foam stability index test. Obstet Gynecol 55:617, 1980.

126. Abromovich DR: The volume of amniotic fluid and its regulating factors. *In* Fairweather DVI, Eskes TKAB (eds): Amniotic Fluid: Research and Clinical Applications. Excerpta Medica, Amsterdam, 1978, p. 31.

127. Emery AEH: Antenatal diagnosis of genetic disease. Mod Trends Hum Genet 1:267, 1970.

128. Queenan JT: When and how to do amniocentesis. Contemp Ob/Gyn 15:61–81, 1980.

129. Verp MS, Gerbie AB, Simpson JL (eds): Antenatal diagnosis of genetic disorders: Amniocentesis for prenatal diagnosis. Clin Obstet Gynecol 24:1007–1021, 1981.

130. Schwarz RH: Amniocentesis. Clin Obstet Gynecol 18:1–22, 1975.

131. Karp LE, Rothwell R, Conrad SH, et al: Ultrasonic placental localization and bloody taps in midtrimester amniocentesis for prenatal genetic diagnosis. Obstet Gynecol 50:589–593, 1977.

132. Hohler CW, Doherty RA, Lea J, et al: Ultrasound placental site in relation to bloody taps in midtrimester amniocentesis. Obstet Gynecol 52:555–557, 1978.

133. Gerbie AB, Elias S: Amniocentesis for antenatal diagnosis of genetic defects. Clin Obstet Gynecol 7:5–12, 1980.
134. Hanson FW, Tennant FR, Zorn EM, et al: Analysis of 2136 genetic amniocenteses: Experience of a single physician. Gynecology 152:436–443, 1985.
135. Kazy Z, Rozovsky IS, Bakharev VA: Chorion biopsy in early pregnancy: A method of early prenatal diagnosis for inherited disorders. Prenat Diagn 2:39–45, 1982.
136. Simoni G, Brambati B, Danesino C, et al: Efficient direct chromosome analyses and enzyme determinations from chorionic villi samples in the first trimester of pregnancy. Hum Genet 63:349–357, 1983.
137. Gosden JR, Mitchell AR, Gosden CM, et al: Direct vision chorionic biopsy and chromosome specific DNA probes for determination of fetal sex in first trimester prenatal diagnosis. Lancet 2:1416–1419, 1982.

Outpatient Arteriography: Visceral and Peripheral Studies

David Dwyer, M.D.

Prior to the mid-1970s, arteriography was considered by most physicians to be an inpatient procedure, necessitating admission to a hospital prior to the study and overnight observation following angiography. However, newer catheters of 3.0 to 5.0 French (F) size, advances in contrast material, and digital subtraction angiography have led to an increasing acceptance of outpatient arteriography for visceral and peripheral examinations. During the past 10 years, a number of radiologists have reported excellent results with outpatient examinations of large groups of patients in diverse clinical settings, ranging from smaller community hospitals to larger centers.[1-6] Virtually any visceral or peripheral angiogram is amenable to an outpatient approach, although the studies most commonly performed include abdominal aortography, selective renal and hepatic arteriography, and pelvic and lower limb angiography.

Cost analyses have shown impressive savings with outpatient studies as compared with inpatient arteriography.[3, 5, 6] The advantages of outpatient examinations are especially compelling for communities where there is a waiting list for hospital admission.[4] In addition, the safety of such an outpatient approach is also well established.[1-6] If complications should arise, the patient can be admitted directly to the hospital. The incidence of such admissions is very low, however, ranging from less than 1% to 6%.[2, 4] Delayed complications such as late bleeding or arterial occlusion are significantly less than 1%.

Outpatient angiography can be performed either in a hospital-based angiography suite or, if available, in an outpatient diagnostic radiologic office or center. If the latter is used, then facilities for observation of patients after angiography must be provided, ideally with a nurse in attendance. This outpatient facility should be located in close proximity to a hospital, where the patient can be admitted for overnight care should the need arise.

PATIENT SELECTION

Patient selection is extremely important for the safety and success of an outpatient angiography program. A physical status classification (developed by the American Society of Anesthesiologists) is shown in Table 7–1. Class I and II patients are successfully handled as outpatients. Severe diabetes, uncontrolled hypertension, borderline renal function, bleeding diathesis, anticoagulant therapy, and end-stage myocardial disease with difficult-to-control congestive heart failure all require hospital admission for arteriography. A history of moderate or severe previous reaction to contrast agents may also be an indication for in-hospital angiography, although such individuals may be treated as outpatients with proper preparation and backup facilities. Finally, the patient must be able to cooperate and follow instructions to comply properly with postprocedure and postdischarge instructions and to be able to recognize specific signs of delayed postprocedure complications. If a patient lives alone, a friend or relative must be able to stay with her or him on the night following the angiogram. Out-of-town patients are directed to stay in a local hotel.

SCHEDULING OF EXAMINATIONS

Ideally, an angiographic procedure is scheduled with the radiologist directly by the referring physician. This permits an accurate communica-

Table 7–1
PHYSICAL STATUS CLASSIFICATION*

Class	Description
I	No organic disease
II	Mild to moderate systemic disease (e.g., mild diabetes, essential hypertension)
III	Severe systemic disease (e.g., severe diabetes, old myocardial infarction)
IV	Constant life-threatening disease (e.g., cardiac insufficiency, pulmonary insufficiency)
V	Moribund

*Developed by the American Society of Anesthesiologists.

tion of patient history, known medical problems, and results of previous examinations and permits the radiologist to ask any necessary questions. As an alternative, a special-procedures technologist or nurse can also be responsible for examination scheduling. Outpatient angiography is most easily performed in the morning so that patients can be discharged from the observation area before the end of the working day. Extensive laboratory work is usually not required in otherwise healthy outpatients scheduled for angiography. However, a recent serum creatinine value should be obtained prior to the patient's appointment for angiography.

It is recommended that the patient be given a set of written instructions prior to coming to the hospital or clinic. These guides can be mailed to the patient at the time the examination is booked, or they can be distributed by the referring physician. Two sample sets of preprocedure instructions are provided here. The instructions in Figure 7–1 are used for in-hospital examinations at Harborview Medical Center, Seattle, Washington. Those in Figure 7–2 are used by a private radiology group in the Seattle area where angiography is performed in a clinic building immediately adjacent to a large hospital. Although the second set of instructions is specifically aimed at a subset of patients undergoing renal digital subtraction studies, it could be successfully adapted to a larger group of outpatient arteriography patients.

To assure that patients have received preangiography instructions, they are contacted by an angiography nurse or technologist by phone 24 hours prior to the angiogram. This procedure gives the patient a chance to ask questions and to be reassured and also ensures that the patient understands the postprocedure protocol. Patients are instructed to take all of their regular medications, especially antihypertensives, with a sip of water on the day of their angiogram. Although insulin adjustments can be handled by the patient's internist or family physician, an acceptable protocol is to have patients administer half of their regular insulin dosage at home before coming in for the angiogram, to administer a 5% dextrose solution at 100 to 120 ml/hour during the angiogram, and then to give the remaining half of the daily insulin dosage postangiography with an early lunch.

EXAMINATION TECHNIQUES

An intravenous line is started prior to angiography as an access route for drug administration, should the need arise. It is left in place until the patient is discharged; although the patient is encouraged to drink fluids during the observation period following the examination, it may be useful to give additional fluids intravenously to ensure adequate hydration. If patients are extremely anxious during the angiogram, 2 to 6 mg of

You have been scheduled for an angiogram on an outpatient basis by Dr. _____.

The date of your angiogram is _____.

You must check in at the Outpatient Registration Desk (Ground South, 9th and Alder

entrance to Harborview Medical Center) at _____

and then report to the Main Radiology Department (Ground Center) at _____.

What is an angiogram? Angiography is a special type of radiology (x-ray) exam that permits your doctors to have pictures of your blood vessels. A tiny plastic tube is inserted into an artery, usually in the region of the groin, and contrast material is injected through the tube as x-rays are taken. After satisfactory pictures are obtained, the tube is withdrawn and you will be sent to the recovery room for 3 to 6 hours for observation before being sent home.

Important Instructions

1. If your angiogram is in the morning, you should have nothing to eat or drink after midnight on the evening before your exam. If your exam is in the afternoon, you may have a clear liquid (coffee, tea, apple juice) breakfast but no solid foods on the day of the angiogram.

No matter when your exam is scheduled, it is very important to take *all* of your regular medications as usual. Even if you are fasting, you can take pills with a sip of water.

If you are diabetic and on insulin, let your doctor know when he or she schedules the angiogram. There will be special instructions pertaining to insulin dosage and calorie intake.

2. Because it will be necessary to avoid activity for 12 hours following the exam, you will not be able to drive home or take a bus after the angiogram. You will need to arrange to have a friend or relative drive you home or accompany you in a taxi and stay with you for at least 6 hours after you arrive home. Because it is difficult to predict how long the test will take, it is best if you plan on calling your friend or relative from the recovery room. Most patients who have an angiogram in the morning are ready to go home by midafternoon. If your test is in the afternoon, you will probably be discharged around dinner time.

Please be on time for your appointment. If you have any questions about the test, feel free to call the angiography nurse (Marcia) at 223-4764.

Figure 7–1. Sample instructions for outpatient angiography.

diazepam can be given intravenously. However, routine sedation is generally not necessary.

Arteriography, using a Seldinger catheter technique, can be performed via femoral, translumbar, or axillary approaches, although a femoral entry site is preferred because of its lower rate of complications.[7] In some cases, such as a single-leg arteriography or a study of arteriovenous dialysis fistulas, angiography is possible directly through the angiographic needle.

The catheter diameter depends on the type of data acquisition being used. If an intraarterial digital subtraction technique is employed, then a 3 F catheter is entirely satisfactory (Fig. 7–3).[8] However, in some cases such as arteriography of the lower extremities or selective visceral angi-

Your physician has referred you to Seattle Radiologists for a Digital Subtraction Angiogram of the renal arteries. This procedure evaluates the blood vessels in your abdomen that supply the kidneys

Our radiologists and highly trained technical staff work with the most advanced computer-assisted equipment. This specialized diagnostic equipment means that we can examine you as an outpatient rather than in a hospital. Our procedure *is more convenient, less time-consuming, less costly*, and because of the computer system it is *considerably more comfortable*.

After processing and developing, your films are interpreted by a board-certified radiologist. A telephone report to your personal physician is available almost immediately, and a written report will be delivered the next day.

PREPARING FOR THE EXAMINATION:

Bowel Preparation

- No solid foods for 24 hours prior to study.
- Two Dulcolax tablets or laxatives of choice by mouth at 7:00 p.m. the evening before.
- A Fleet's enema before bedtime the night before.
- Clear liquids *only* after 12:00 midnight. *Do* drink plenty of fluids.
- A Fleet's enema the morning of the study. (The above medications are nonprescription)

You may take your regular medication the morning of the examination unless your doctor orders otherwise. It is important that you drink plenty of fluids. Fluids are necessary because the "dye" used in the examination can cause an increase in the urine output, and this fluid needs to be replaced. Plan on spending at least 4 to 6 hours in our office.

Following an interview with our nurse, you will go to the preparation room, where you will disrobe and put on a gown. An IV (intravenous) will be started to give you medication if needed as well as additional fluids. You will then go to the DSA room for the examination.

DSA EXAMINATION:

A small area in your groin will be shaved, cleansed thoroughly, and covered with sterile drapes. Using local anesthesia, the radiologist will numb a small area. A very small plastic tube called a catheter will then be inserted into the blood vessel and appropriately positioned. A special contrast (dye) will then be injected through the tube to opacify the blood vessels, and a series of x-ray exposures will be made. A digital computer coupled to the x-ray detectors will then analyze the image. The computer brings out information in the image that would not otherwise be visible to the eye. The attending radiologist reviews the images and then prepares a written report for your doctor.

A radiologist, x-ray technologist, and a nurse will be present throughout the examination. You will feel minimum discomfort during this procedure, but expect to experience a warm flushed feeling in your abdomen each time the contrast (dye) is injected. This sensation goes away within seconds. Your cooperation will be asked for in breath holding and in positioning.

FOLLOWING THE EXAMINATION:

The catheter will be removed and pressure held upon the groin for approximately 10 to 15 minutes. You will then be sent to a recovery area and observed for at least 4 hours. You will be asked to keep your leg still during this time. Lunch and further liquids will be available. During the recovery period, you will be routinely monitored by the nursing staff.

When your renal angiogram is completed, you are to *be escorted home by a relative or friend because you will not be able to drive a vehicle*. Please follow these instructions closely:

- Continue to drink plenty of fluids (at least 8 oz. every hour until bedtime).
- Do not engage in any strenuous physical activity, and avoid any rapid motion.
- You may continue taking any prescribed medications.
- Avoid hot baths for 24 hours.

Staff are on duty at the Nordstrom office between 8:00 a.m. and 5:50 p.m. to answer any questions you may have about the DSA examination. You can reach the office at 292-6233. There is little chance that problems will occur, but you should report any of the following:

- Continued bleeding
- Swelling over the site of the needle puncture
- Redness and/or tenderness up your leg
- Any other unusual symptoms

After hours questions: Call 386-2241, where a radiologist is on call.

Figure 7–2. Sample instructions for patients undergoing renal digital subtraction studies.

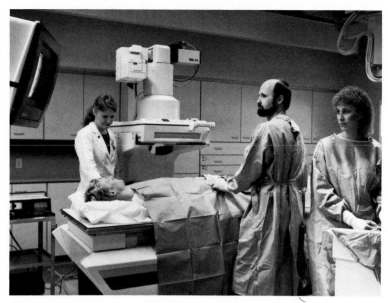

Figure 7–3. Digital subtraction technique can often be used for a majority of the necessary filming during angiography.

ography, conventional cut-film arteriography may be desirable. Therefore, a 4 or 5 F catheter is necessary to accommodate the higher-volume injections of more viscous contrast material. Additional views of distal vessels or oblique projections can be accomplished using digital subtraction as an adjunct, thereby reducing the overall contrast requirements.

POSTANGIOGRAPHIC CARE

Following angiography, patients are observed either in a special area in the radiology department or in an outpatient recovery room. Nursing orders are similar to those written for inpatient angiography, with a provision for frequent arteriotomy site checks, as well as for the observation of distal pulses and vital signs. Oral fluid intake is encouraged to maintain hydration. After 4 hours, the patient is ambulated under observation and then discharged to home with an instruction sheet (Fig. 7–4). Among other things, this sheet emphasizes the need for bed rest for the remainder of the day and describes techniques to deal with delayed bleeding. Should the patient have questions, the hospital telephone number (as well as the name of the angiographer and referring physician) is noted on the instruction sheet.

You have had the following procedure: _____

_____ .

Your doctors' names are: _____

You may call 223-3010 (Harborview Paging Operator) to reach your doctor if you have questions or concerns. If your physician is not on-call, the operator will contact the appropriate on-call doctor for you. If for some reason the operator cannot locate the doctor for you and you have concerns regarding your condition, have someone bring you to the Harborview Emergency Room.

PLEASE FOLLOW THESE IMPORTANT INSTRUCTIONS:

1. Following angiography, it is very important to let the small hole in your groin artery heal completely. To ensure that there is no bleeding from this small hole:

Do not walk or stand any more than is absolutely necessary for 12 hours after you get home from the hospital. Either spend the rest of the day in an easy chair or in bed.

If there is any bleeding or swelling at your groin, it is important to have someone compress it firmly; this compression is done by placing all four fingers over the hole and pressing straight down. Call your doctor right away. You should also call your doctor immediately if either foot becomes painful.

2. During the angiogram, radiographic contrast material (dye) was injected into your arteries. This is removed from your bloodstream by the kidneys. To help flush this dye out of your system, it is very important to drink lots of liquid (water, juice, coffee, or tea) on the day following the test—a glass of water every hour during the afternoon and evening after your angiogram would be ideal.

3. On the day following your angiogram, you may resume normal activity and remove the small Band-Aid from your groin. We would recommend against strenous activity (running, heavy housework, etc.) for two to three days.

4. If your Harborview doctor has not talked with you in the recovery room, you should call his or her office in the next few days to receive instructions about follow-up appointments.

Figure 7–4. Sample outpatient postangiography instructions.

ANGIOPLASTY

The preprocedure workup for angioplasty is more extensive than that for routine angiography. To ensure that effective postangioplasty follow-up can be performed, patients should be screened by a vascular surgeon, and Doppler pulse pressures should be recorded.

The efficacy of percutaneous transluminal angioplasty has been well established. It is often performed at the time of initial pelvic or peripheral arteriography, with a catheter already in the arterial system traversing a stenosis. The possibility of angioplasty can be discussed with the referring vascular surgeon at the time of angiography scheduling. If angioplasty is anticipated, informed consent can be obtained from the patient at the same time as consent for angiography. Alternatively, angioplasty can be performed as a second procedure. The advantage of this latter approach is that the patient's referring vascular surgeon and diagnostic radiologist are able to discuss therapeutic alternatives, avoiding a single lengthy combined procedure with its associated increased contrast dosage.

In one recent series of 75 consecutive patients who had transluminal angioplasty performed on an outpatient basis, only 2 necessitated hospital admission as the result of arterial reocclusion.[9] A third patient was readmitted 18 hours after the angiogram because of an unspecified contrast reaction. There were no major complications in another series of 70 peripheral angioplasties in 64 patients.[10] A single patient was admitted to the hospital for a suspected false aneurysm. In a telephone survey of this second series of patients, 99% were satisfied with the outpatient approach to angioplasty. In both series, patients were discharged 4 to 6 hours after angioplasty if they were stable and in satisfactory condition, with home care instructions as previously described in this chapter.

As discussed by Redman in a recent commentary article, a reasonable estimate of peripheral transluminal angioplasty complication rate is 2 to 3%, with the vast majority of these complications occurring during the procedure or in the immediate postprocedure period.[11] Iliac and femoral angioplasties are the most amenable to outpatient treatment; renal and tibiopopliteal dilatation are probably best handled as inpatient procedures in most centers. In conclusion, radiologists and vascular surgeons are more likely to consider angioplasty as an outpatient procedure because of smaller 5 F diameter angioplasty catheters, increasing experience with angioplasty by many radiologists, and published series of successful outpatient angioplasties.

SUMMARY

Outpatient arteriography is possible for most patients undergoing visceral and peripheral angiography, provided there is close consultation between the radiologist and referring physician, thoughtful patient screening, and well-organized pre- and postprocedure patient care. As an extension of arteriography, outpatient angioplasty shows promise, further reducing patient-care costs without compromising the efficacy or safety of this procedure.

References

1. Giustra PE, Killoran AD: Outpatient arteriography at a small community hospital. Radiology 116:581–583, 1975.
2. Taheri SA, Sheehan FR: Translumbar aortography as an outpatient procedure (Letter). AJR 137:1287, 1981.
3. Rogers W, Mothart RW: Outpatient arteriography and cardiac catheterization: Effective alternatives to inpatient procedures. AJR 144:233–234, 1985.

4. Saint-Georges G, Aube M: Safety of outpatient angiography: A prospective study. AJR 144:235–236, 1985.
5. Adams PS, Roub LW: Outpatient angiography and interventional radiology: Safety and cost benefits. Radiology, 151:81–82, 1984.
6. Wolfel DA, Lovett BP, Ortenburger AI, et al: Outpatient arteriography: Its safety and cost effectiveness. Radiology 153:363–364, 1984.
7. Hessel SJ, Adams DF, Abrams HL: Complications of angiography. Radiology 138:273–281, 1981.
8. Bunker SR, Cutaia FI, Fritz AL, et al: Femoral interarterial digital angiography: An outpatient procedure. AJR 141:593–596, 1983.
9. Manashil GB, Thunstrom BS, Thorpe CD, et al: Outpatient transluminal angioplasty. Radiology 147:7–8, 1983.
10. Lemarbre L, Hudon L, Coche G, et al: Outpatient peripheral angioplasty: Survey of complications and patients' perceptions. AJR 148:1239–1240, 1987.
11. Redman H: Commentary: Has the time come for outpatient peripheral angioplasty? AJR 148:1241–1242, 1987.

CHAPTER 8

Digital Subtraction Angiography of the Heart and the Thoracic Vessels

Hugo G. Bogren, M.D.

Recent developments in cardiac angiography have altered the traditional practice of cardiac radiology. These advances include the use of outpatient facilities for cardiac studies, the introduction of nonionic contrast agents, and the use of intravenous and intraarterial digital subtraction angiography (DSA).

Mahrer and Eshoo evaluated outpatient conventional cine cardiac catheterization in more than 1,800 patients, the majority of whom underwent left heart and coronary angiography.[1] There was quite a low complication rate and only one death, comparable to the complication rates reported in the literature.[1] The estimated savings (compared with inpatient angiography) were $334,000, based on 1,000 catheterizations per year (70% outpatients). Fierens reported more than 5,000 outpatient coronary angiographies using the Sones technique, cineangiography, and the brachial artery approach, with a resultant 2% complication rate and no deaths.[2] Fierens calculated a possible annual savings of more than $78,000,000 per year by performing coronary angiography on an outpatient basis, assuming 300,000 coronary angiograms in the United States per year (75% outpatients).[2] Baird, Beauchamp, and Rogers and colleagues have confirmed the safety and economic advantage of outpatient catheterization.[3-5]

Newer nonionic contrast agents appear to have fewer cardiac side effects than conventional ionic materials.[6-8] These effects include a lowered sensation of heat and a slightly decreased degree of toxicity. However, the nonionic agents are quite expensive compared with ionic materials,

125

limiting the acceptance of these newer substances (see Chapter 3). DSA can reduce the amounts of both ionic and nonionic contrast agents necessary for cardiac evaluation.

DSA has been widely used to visualize peripheral arteries since the equipment became commercially available in 1980–81. Cardiac applications were attempted at the same time and were successful in ischemic heart disease to evaluate left ventricular volume and function.[9, 10] The evaluation of more detailed cardiac or vascular pathology in the thorax, such as congenital heart disease, requires more refined techniques. The latter have recently become possible using ECG gating and short pulse-width acquisition. Although not yet widely used, outpatient DSA may now be used in a variety of cardiac and great vessel malformations if the proper technique is applied. In general, DSA provides an almost instantaneous review of collected images, thereby improving the quality and decreasing the time of each individual examination.

Because of cardiac contractions, respiration, and the need for rapid acquisition rates, cardiac applications require more sophisticated hardware and software than does peripheral angiography. The special technique for acquiring and processing high-resolution digital cardiac images will therefore be described in some detail.

TECHNICAL ASPECTS

ECG Gating

The application of the subtraction process to cardiovascular structures is complicated by periodic variations in background density caused by cardiac contractions. To eliminate errors due to cardiac motion, background images from the same phase of the cardiac cycle as the contrast images should be used as subtraction masks. This requires ECG gating as illustrated in Figure 8–1.[11, 12] ECG gating is relatively easy to perform by integrating the ECG signal with images acquired by the computer. Attempts have been made to eliminate noise from cardiac motion by the use of a mask obtained by averaging up to 30 images from one cardiac cycle, but this technique is less effective than precise ECG gating.[13]

Respiratory Gating

The error in the subtraction process caused by respiratory motion is a more serious problem than image degradation caused by a cardiac movement. The heart, pulmonary and great vessels, diaphragm, and ribs all move during respiration, causing large artifacts if respiration is not

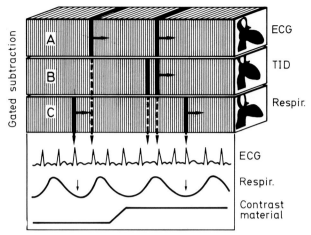

Figure 8–1. Image-acquisition techniques in digital angiocardiography. **A**, ECG gating; **B**, time interval differencing **(TID)**. **C**, respiration gating.

completely stopped or gated.[14] Most adults and older children are able to hold their breath, but infants and small children cannot stop respiration on command. Since a large number of patients with congenital heart disease are very young and many patients with ischemic heart disease are very sick, respiratory motion, if not compensated for, is perhaps the most important factor limiting the use of digital angiocardiography in these patient groups.

Smaller respiratory motion artifacts may be eliminated by pixel shifting, but if recording occurs during respiration, gating must be applied. Respiratory gating (Fig. 8–1) has been used successfully in experimental situations employing a method designed by Brennecke and colleagues.[15] The combination of ECG and respiratory gating may be difficult, but in normal breathing the end-inspiration phase is often long enough for the same ECG phase to be chosen also (Fig. 8–1). Other techniques that can be attempted are subtraction of opacified right from left heart frames and a trial-and-error method using different masks.[16, 17]

Short Pulse-Width Acquisition

Cineangiocardiography typically uses 60 frames/second, pulsed radiation, and pulse-widths of 2 to 5 msec. Longer pulse-widths cause motion unsharpness in the images. Short pulse-width acquisition requires that the DSA equipment be capable of progressive readout of the TV camera target.[18] Although some manufacturers now supply such progressive readouts, most units still read the TV camera target in an interlaced mode that requires a 33- to 150-msec pulse-width. A comparison between the interlaced (33-msec pulse-width) and progressive readout (5-msec pulse-width) is demonstrated in Figure 8–2. Figure 8–2*A* (progressive readout) shows better edge detection and higher resolution (as evidenced by visualization of the coronary arteries), as compared with Figure 8–2*B* (interlaced readout). The left circumflex artery is seen as it runs in the atrial ventricular groove, thereby identifying the plane of the mitral valve. Identification of the mitral valve is necessary for the determination of accurate ventricular volume and ejection fraction. However, the latter is difficult to achieve if 33-msec pulse-width and interlaced readout are used.

X-Ray Dose

A high signal-to-noise ratio must be obtained to produce adequate images. This ratio can be increased by various means; the least complex method uses an increased radiation dose. This method is used in most applications in peripheral angiography when only 1 to 2 images/second are needed, with a resultant skin dose of 200 mR per image. However, in angiocardiography with 30 frames/second, low-dose radiography is mandatory. In the latter circumstance, the signal-to-noise ratio can be increased by averaging images, thereby allowing a smaller x-ray dose per image. The use of 4.5 mm of aluminum filtration in digital angiocardiography reduces the skin dose by 25%, while the effective imaging dose is much less reduced with maintained signal-to-noise ratio and contrast resolution. A matrix of 256 × 256 is adequate for ventricular studies if 30 frames/second are recorded. If the matrix is changed to 512 × 512 and if the same signal-to-noise ratio per pixel is to be maintained, the radiation dose is increased by a factor of four. Since low frame rates reduce the dose, we often use ECG-gated images per cardiac cycle after intravenous injection to evaluate cardiac chambers and the thoracic aorta. If such a low frame rate is employed, then the matrix can be increased to 512 × 512. A simple rule of thumb is not to use more x-rays per run than in cineangiocardiography. A typical cine technique is 65 to 85 kV and 1 mAs at 60 frames/second. With DSA, this dose can be maintained or increased in proportion to the lower frame rate. At less than 30 frames/second, progressive readout of the TV camera target lowers the dose three times more.[18]

Choice of Projection in Intravenous Digital Angiocardiography

Ischemic Heart Disease. The most commonly used cineangiocardiography projection to evaluate left ventricular volume and function in ischemic heart disease is the 30-degree right anterior oblique (RAO) projection.

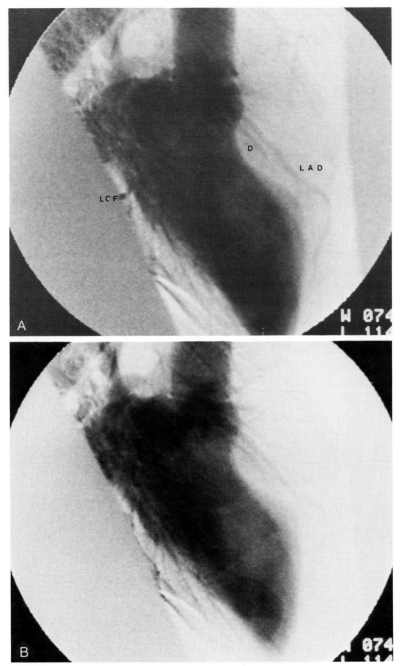

Figure 8–2. Left ventricular angiogram of a 46-kg dog after superior vena cava injection of 30 ml of 76% Renografin. Both images were ECG gated. *(A)* Progressive readout with 5 msec pulse-width. *(B)* Interlaced mode with 33-msec pulse width. **LAD,** left anterior descending coronary artery; **D,** diagonal branch; **LCF,** left circumflex artery.

From the data obtained, left ventricular volume is computed using Dodge's area-length method in a single plane. This also appears to be the projection of choice for intravenous digital angiocardiography in ischemic heart disease. The four-chamber digital view originally described for use in congenital heart disease by Bargeron and colleagues has great advantages in intravenous angiocardiography, as there is no superimposition of chambers with this projection.[19, 20] Als and associates used this view in a biplane method and found it more accurate than ordinary RAO–LAO biplane for ventricular volume and function evaluation.[21] Lipton and colleagues showed that the single-plane method using the angulated view and Simpson's rule was more accurate than biplane methods.[22]

Congenital Heart Disease. The four-chamber view originally developed by Bargeron and associates is the ideal view for intravenous angiocardiography in congenital heart disease.[19, 20] It not only eliminates superposition of cardiac chambers, but is also one of the most useful views in the diagnosis of congenital heart disease.[23] Figure 8–3 displays video densograms with recordings from the left and right cardiac chambers. Contrast medium was injected into the patient's antecubital vein. Some contrast medium remains in the right ventricle during the passage of the contrast medium through the left ventricle. Separation of the four chambers is especially important when attempting to quantitate ventricular ejection fraction or left-to-right shunts using time/density curves, a technique currently being developed. An illustration of the four-chamber views in congenital heart disease is seen in Figure 8–4.

Injection Technique

In adult patients and older children, we recommend injection into the right atrium. Peripheral injections and injection in the superior or inferior vena cava have been used, but the best bolus is obtained if the medium is injected directly into the right atrium.

In infants and small children, we usually use peripheral injections into the left femoral vein (which is larger than the arm veins). Because the distance from the femoral vein to the heart in children is small compared with that in adults, a satisfactory bolus is obtained using this technique. Flushing with saline following the contrast injection may improve the bolus of contrast material. An efficient way to flush is to contain all the contrast medium in a plastic tubing of adequate length, and then use a power injector filled with saline to propel the contrast medium into the vein.[17]

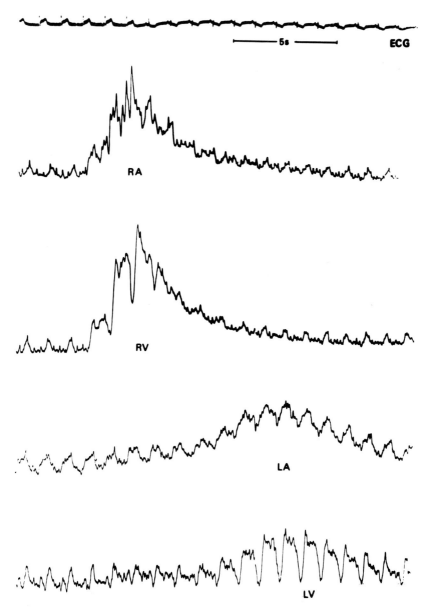

Figure 8–3. Time/density curves from a patient studied in the four-chamber view after peripheral vein injection. **RA,** right atrium; **RV,** right ventricle; **LA,** left atrium; **LV,** left ventricle. (From Bogren HG, Bürsch JH: Digital angiography in the diagnosis of congenital heart disease. Cardiovasc Intervent Radiol 7:180–188, 1984.)

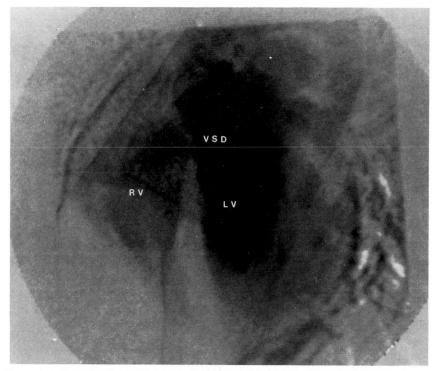

Figure 8–4. Four-chamber DSA image obtained after injection of 10 ml of Angiovist 370 in the right iliac vein of a four-year-old girl with ventricular septal defect **(VSD). LV,** left ventricle; **RV,** right ventricle.

CLINICAL STUDIES

Ischemic Heart Disease

Clinical applications in ischemic heart disease for the quantitation of left ventricular dimensions and function have been performed systematically by Tobis and colleagues, Higgins and associates, and many others.[9–10, 24–25] All investigators have used x-ray fluoroscopy with 33-msec pulse-width, but the resolution of the images has not always been optimal. DSA left ventricular volume and ejection fraction determinations have been accurately performed and compare favorably with the results obtained by direct cineventriculography. DSA exercise studies and the intravenous injection of contrast medium have been performed following bicycle stress testing or after right atrial pacing.[26, 27]

Left ventricular volume and ejection fraction determinations are easy to perform and do not necessarily require high-resolution images with the use of short pulse-width and progressive readout. In the future, it is expected that more detailed information about left ventricular function, wall motion, and morphology will be obtained using ECG gating and short pulse-width acquisition. A recent example from our laboratory is seen in Figure 8–5.

Aortic Aneurysm or Dissection

Intravenous DSA aortography following aortic dissection repair can be performed on outpatients.[28] Intravenous and intraarterial DSA aortography in acute dissections has also been performed, but patients are generally severely ill and thus these examinations are best undertaken in a hospital setting. Aortic aneurysms, both traumatic and arteriosclerotic, can also be evaluated by DSA.[29–30]

Congenital Heart Disease

Intravenous DSA in outpatients with suspected congenital heart disease is useful. One common indication for DSA is the evaluation of congenital abnormalities of the aorta and aortic arch.[31] An example of an aberrant left subclavian artery in a child with a right aortic arch is seen in Figure 8–6. This patient was originally thought to have a vascular ring, but the DSA diagnosis made surgical correction and hospitalization unnecessary. Figure 8–7 shows an example of coarctation of the aorta. This patient was a 14-year-old boy who had a pressure difference of 40 mm Hg between the arms and legs and who underwent echocardiography and outpatient digital DSA. Echocardiography showed only a tricuspid aortic valve, but the digital study showed a classic aortic coarctation with a mildly narrowed prestenotic segment and a normal-sized poststenotic region. An example of a minor coarctation is illustrated in Figure 8–8. Note the excellent demonstration of the vertebral artery originating from the aortic arch. The coarctation was mild, and surgery was not indicated.

The Cleveland Clinic has the largest experience in intravenous DSA in congenital heart disease.[31] Most of their studies were on inpatients, since the intravenous DSA studies had to be verified by hospital-based cardiac catheterization. Some congenital heart lesions are suitable for outpatient intravenous DSA, such as postoperative follow-up studies, but the indications are still somewhat unclear. We have also used DSA to verify a Blalock-Taussig anastomosis and to evaluate the growth of the pulmonary artery following shunt operation for pulmonary atresia. The Cleveland Clinic has attempted to quantitate left-to-right shunts from time/density curves in patients with atrial and septal defects.[32] In 10 of 10 cases, an atrial septal defect (ASD) was identified, but only 6 of 9 patients

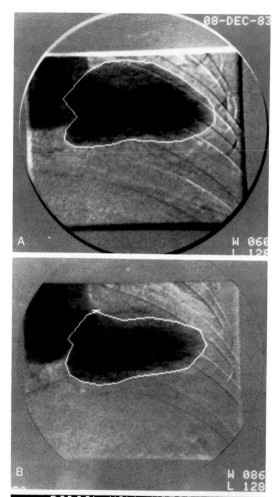

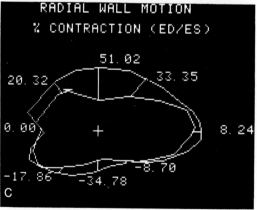

Figure 8–5. Left ventriculogram after IV injection in a patient with inferior wall myocardial infarction. *(A)* End diastole. *(B)* End systole. *(C)* Ejection fraction and wall motion analysis. Ejection fraction was computer calculated to 38%.

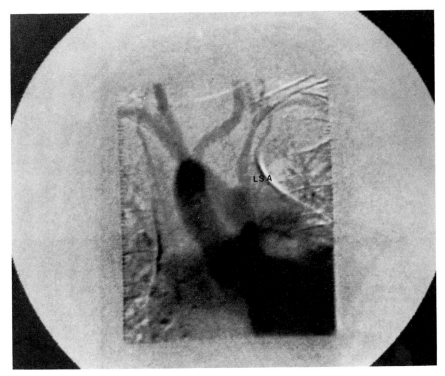

Figure 8–6. Right aortic arch and aberrant left subclavian artery **(LSA)**. DSA image in AP projection after femoral vein injection of 7.5 ml of Angiovist 370 in a 15-month-old child.

with ventricular septal defect (VSD) were correctly diagnosed. We have shown experimentally (using a method to quantitate left-to-right shunts by time/density curves), that ASD, VSD, and patent ductus arteriosus (PDA) defects can be diagnosed with DSA in shunts of approximately 1.5 to 1 (Fig. 8–4).[33] This technique should increase the indications for intravenous cardiac DSA, and particularly shunt determinations in patients with left-to-right flow defects. Since the natural history of many VSDs is to close spontaneously, outpatient intravenous DSA is particularly suited for follow-up studies in such individuals.

Another center with considerable experience in congenital heart disease is the University of Kiel, in West Germany.[17, 34] Practitioners there have performed approximately 35 outpatient DSA studies in children with suspected functional murmurs and have obtained excellent clinical or surgical correlation. They have also performed a large number of post-surgical follow-up studies.

We have performed outpatient DSA using aortic injection in three children with Kawasaki disease. A small catheter and a supravalvular intraarterial injection clearly demonstrated the extent of coronary artery

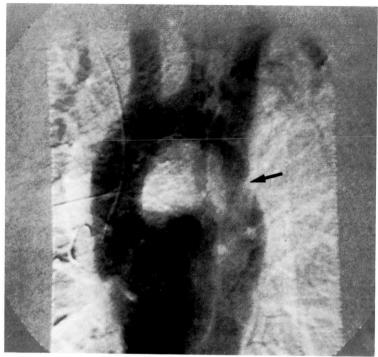

Figure 8–7. Coarctation of the aorta. DSA angiogram in a 14-year-old boy weighing 50 kg after injection of 25 ml of Angiovist 370 into the right atrium. The moderately severe coarctation is well seen (arrow).

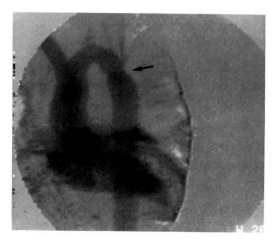

Figure 8–8. Subtraction image after injection of 12 ml 76% Renografin in the right atrium of a 6-year-old girl with minimal coarction. The small coarctation is seen (arrow), as well as the separate origin of the left vertebral artery.

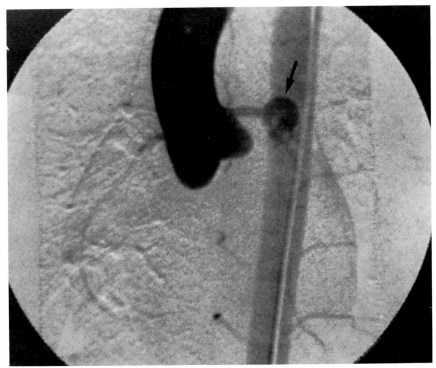

Figure 8–9. Twelve ml of Angiovist 370 was injected into the ascending aorta and ECG-gated two images per cycle were recorded digitally. A large aneurysm (arrow) of the left anterior descending coronary artery with very poor runoff is present. This 8-year-old boy (25 kg) had Kawasaki disease.

aneurysms in these patients (Fig. 8–9). After the conclusion of the study, the patients were kept in the hospital and surveyed for complications for 4 hours, and then they were sent home.

To summarize the use of outpatient DSA in congenital heart disease, clear-cut indications are aortic arch anomalies and postoperative follow-up studies. Another indication may be suspected functional murmurs and follow-up studies in closing VSDs. If left-to-right shunt determinations become successful, a whole new field of congenital heart disease will be open for outpatient intravenous DSA. Recent legislation, particularly in the State of California, has authorized full-fledged and pilot projects for the operation and development of outpatient cardiac catheterization laboratories.[35] DSA has been recommended as an alternative to cineangiography and should further spur the growth and usefulness of this technique in the evaluation of cardiac disease.

References

1. Mahrer PR, Eshoo N: Outpatient cardiac catheterization and coronary angiography. Cathet Cardiovasc Diagn 7:355–360, 1981.

2. Fierens E: Outpatient coronary arteriography. Cathet Cardiovasc Diagn 10:27–32, 1984.
3. Baird CL: Ambulatory cardiac catheterization. Va Med 107:621–622, 1980.
4. Beauchamp PX: Ambulatory cardiac catheterization cuts costs for hospitals and patients. Hospital 1:62–63, 1981.
5. Rogers WF, Moothart RW: Outpatient arteriography and cardiac catheterization: Effective alternatives to inpatient procedures. AJR 144:233–234, 1985.
6. Higgins CB: Overview of cardiovascular effects of contrast media. Comparison of ionic and nonionic media. Invest Radiol 5:187–190, 1984.
7. Salem DN, Koustam MA, Isner JM, et al: Comparison of effects on left ventricular ejection fraction of iopamidol and renografin during left ventriculography and coronary arteriography. Invest Radiol 5:203–205, 1984.
8. Cuiffo AA, Fuchs RM, Guzman PA, et al: Benefits of nonionic contrast in coronary arteriography. Preliminary results of a randomized double-blind trial comparing iopamidol with renografin-76. Invest Radiol 5:197–202, 1984.
9. Tobis J, Nalcioglu O, Johnston WD, et al: Left ventricular imaging with digital subtraction angiography using intravenous contrast injection and fluoroscopic exposure levels. Am Heart J 104:20–27, 1982.
10. Higgins CB, Norris SL, Gerber KH, et al: Quantitation of left ventricular dimensions and function by digital video subtraction angiography. Radiology 144:461–469, 1982.
11. Brennecke R, Brown TK, Bürsch JH, et al: Digital processing of videoangiocardiographic image series using a minicomputer. Proceedings from Computers in Cardiology, IEEE Catalog No. 76CH1160-IC, 1976, pp 255–260.
12. Brennecke R, Brown TK, Bürsch JH, et al: Computerized video-image preprocessing with applications to cardioangiographic roentgen-image series. In Nagel HH (ed): Digital Image Processing. Springer-Verlag, Berlin, 1977, pp 244–262.
13. Kruger RA, Mistretta CA, Houk TL, et al: Computerized fluoroscopy techniques for intravenous study of cardiac chamber dynamics. Invest Radiol 14:279–287, 1979.
14. Bogren HG, Lantz BMT, Miller RR, et al: Effect of respiration on cardiac motion determined by cineangiography. Acta Radiol Diagn 18:609–620, 1977.
15. Brennecke R, Hahne HJ, Moldenhauer K, et al: Improved digital real-time processing and storage techniques with applications to intravenous contrast angiography. Computers in Cardiology, IEEE Catalog No. 78 CH1391-2, 1978, pp 191–194.
16. Bogren HG, Bürsch JH, Brennecke R, et al: Intravenous angiocardiography using digital image processing. I. Experience with axial projections in normal pigs. Invest Radiol 17:216–223, 1982.
17. Bogren HG, Bürsch JH: Digital angiography in the diagnosis of congenital heart disease. Cardiovasc Intervent Radiol 7:180–188, 1984.
18. Bogren HG, Seibert JA, Hines HH, et al: The beneficial effects of short pulse width acquisition and ECG-gating in digital angiocardiography. Invest Radiol 19:284–290, 1984.
19. Bargeron LM Jr, Elliott LP, Soto B, et al: Axial cineangiography in congenital heart disease: Section I. Concept, technical and anatomic considerations. Circulation 56:1075–1083, 1977.
20. Elliott LP, Bargeron LM Jr, Beam PR, et al: Axial cineangiography in congenital heart disease: Section II. Specific lesions. Circulation 56:1084–1093, 1977.
21. Als AV, Paulin S, Aroesty JM: Biplane angiographic volumetry using the right anterior oblique and half-axial left anterior oblique technique. Radiology 126:511–514, 1978.
22. Lipton MJ, Hayashi TT, Davis PL, et al: The effects of orientation on volume measurements of human left ventricular casts. Invest Radiol 15:469, 1980.
23. Bogren HG, Bürsch JH, Brennecke R, et al: Choice of projection in intravenous digital angiocardiography. In Heintzen PH, Brennecke R (eds): Digital Imaging in Cardiovascular Radiology. Georg Thieme Verlag, Stuttgart, 1983, pp 212–214.
24. Engels PHC, Ludwig JW, Verhoeven LAJ: Left ventricle evaluation by digital video subtraction angiocardiography. Radiology 144:471–474, 1982.

25. Goldberg HL, Borer JS, Moses JW, et al: Digital subtraction intravenous left ventricular angiography: Comparison with conventional intraventricular angiography. J Am Coll Cardiol 1:858–862, 1983.

26. Johnson RA, Wasserman AG, Leiboff RH, et al: Intravenous digital left ventriculography at rest and with atrial pacing as a screening procedure for coronary artery disease. J Am Coll Cardiol 2:905–910, 1983.

27. Goldberg HL, Moses JW, Borer JS, et al: Exercise left ventriculography utilizing intravenous digital angiography. J Am Coll Cardiol 2:1092–1098, 1983.

28. Guthaner DF, Brody WR, Miller DC: Intravenous aortography after aortic dissection repair. AJR 137:1019–1022, 1981.

29. Moodie DS, Yiannikas J, Gill CC, et al: Intravenous digital subtraction angiography in the evaluation of congenital abnormalities of the aorta and aortic arch. Am Heart J 104:628–634, 1982.

30. Mirvis SE, Pais SO, Gens DR: Thoracic aortic rupture: Advantages of intra-arterial digital subtraction angiography. AJR 146:987–991, 1986.

31. Buonocore E, Pavlicek W, Modic MT, et al: Anatomic and functional imaging of congenital heart disease with digital subtraction angiography. Radiology 147:647–654, 1983.

32. Yiannikas J, Moodie DS, Gill CC, et al: Intravenous digital subtraction angiography in the assessment of patients with left to right shunts before and after surgical correction. J Am Coll Cardiol 3:1507–1514, 1984.

33. Bogren HG, Bürsch JH, Brennecke R, et al: Intravenous angiocardiography using digital image processing: II. Detection of left-to-right shunts in an animal model. Invest Radiol 18:11–17, 1983.

34. Bürsch JH, Brennecke R, Radtke W, et al: Digital fluorography: Applications in congenital heart disease. *In* Heintzen PH, Brennecke R (eds): Digital Imaging in Cardiovascular Radiology. Georg Thieme Verlag, Stuttgart, 1983, pp 216–225.

35. California State Senate Bill SB 554, 1985.

CHAPTER 9

Outpatient CT-Guided Percutaneous Needle Biopsy Techniques

David Dwyer, M.D.

One of the most useful interventional procedures currently being performed in many radiology departments is computed tomography (CT)-guided percutaneous needle biopsy.[1-3] The lung, liver, pancreas, renal cysts, and retroperitoneal masses or lymph nodes are most commonly biopsied. The value of percutaneous biopsy is well established. Accuracy rates vary from 60 to 98%, depending on the specific biopsy site as well as the expertise of the radiologists and pathologist.[2]

Because of the low rate of serious or late complications from needle biopsy, this procedure is well suited to an outpatient approach. In a comprehensive review of the literature, as well as in a large survey of multiple medical centers, Smith collated a series of 63,108 fine-needle aspiration biopsies using 20- to 23-gauge needles.[1] There were four deaths (an incidence of 0.006%), three from hemorrhage and one very indirectly attributed to the biopsy that occurred 6 weeks after biopsy during surgery. Hemorrhage occurred in 0.4% and bile leak in 0.08% of the patients. Infection was rare (0.03%), and needle tract seeding of tumor cells following fine-needle biopsy was documented in only three cases (0.005%). Although the definition of "fine needle" varies from author to author, a 22-gauge needle is the most widely used caliber. This needle size is adequate for obtaining satisfactory amounts of tissue and is also safe for virtually all biopsy procedures, including those in which the biopsy route traverses lung, solid or hollow organs in the abdomen, and vascular structures (including major veins such as inferior vena cava or hilar vessels, although ideally the needle route should try to avoid these areas).

Table 9–1
INDICATIONS FOR BIOPSY WITH CT GUIDANCE

Adrenal mass
Retroperitoneal organs (pancreas) and lymph nodes
Intrathoracic masses close to vascular structures—hilar and mediastinal areas
Intrahepatic lesions not easily seen on ultrasonography
Lung masses not easily seen fluoroscopically

CT VERSUS OTHER IMAGING MODALITIES

The techniques of needle biopsy have been thoroughly explained in standard interventional radiology texts, as well as in excellent review articles in radiology literature.[2] CT, ultrasonography, or fluoroscopy can be used as guidance, depending on the location and size of the lesion and preference of the radiologist. In general, large intraabdominal masses, including intrahepatic lesions, pancreatic masses, and renal cysts with indeterminate echogenicity, are most easily handled with ultrasound-guided needle placement because of the speed and relative ease of this technique. Intrathoracic lesions, especially those in the lung parenchyma that are visible fluoroscopically, are best approached under direct fluoroscopic guidance, ideally in a radiology suite equipped with a C arm or biplane fluoroscopic equipment. Smaller lesions, including adrenal masses, retroperitoneal lymph nodes at least 2 to 3 cm in diameter, intrahepatic or pancreatic masses not easily seen with ultrasonography, and small intrathoracic masses or those located adjacent to major structures in the hilar or mediastinal areas, are best approached by CT-guided biopsy (Table 9–1).

PATIENT SCHEDULING

Biopsies are ideally scheduled directly with a radiologist who can decide which method of guidance will be used. The referring physician should provide any previous diagnostic studies prior to the time scheduled for biopsy, thereby avoiding last-minute deliberation or change of plans. Unless the patient has a bleeding diathesis, has hepatic or renal dysfunction, or other clinical suspicion of thrombocytopenia, extensive prebiopsy laboratory work is usually not necessary.

Relative contraindications to needle biopsy include bleeding diathesis or the inability of the patient to cooperate. Echinococcal cysts have traditionally been regarded as an absolute contraindication to biopsy because of the risk of cyst rupture with seeding of daughter cysts, as well as the possibility of anaphylaxis from the introduction of antigenic cyst contents into the bloodstream. However, 11 hydatid cyst aspirations were included in one series, with no reported complications.[1] Contraindications to lung biopsy include pulmonary hypertension, arteriovenous malformations, and severe chronic obstructive pulmonary disease.

TECHNIQUE

In most patients scheduled for CT-guided biopsy, preliminary CT will have been performed (which demonstrates the mass or other lesion to be approached). The preferable biopsy route is one in which the needle tract is along an axial plane (i.e., entirely within one CT image). This avoids complex angulation of the needle. Otherwise, the most direct route with an attempt to avoid major vascular structures should be selected. If a tract perpendicular to the skin surface is possible, it usually simplifies the biopsy. For lesions in the retroperitoneum or posterior thorax, a posterior approach with the patient prone is preferred.

Using the CT scout image (as well as the patient's previous CT examination for orientation), 5-mm-thick contiguous images are obtained through the region of interest with the patient positioned as he or she will be for the biopsy. Six to eight images are usually adequate to localize the biopsy level. The technologist can then use a skin marking pen to indicate the axial level chosen by the radiologist (Fig. 9–1). The skin entry site for the biopsy needle is then marked with reference to a landmark easily seen on both CT image and the patient. For example, for a retroperitoneal lymph node biopsy via a posterior approach, the vertebral body spinous process is used as a midline indicator and the needle entry site is measured laterally from this point (Fig. 9–2). If there is any doubt about landmarks, a small 1- to 2-cm length of plastic tubing can be taped longitudinally to the patient's skin at the expected needle entry site and an additional CT image obtained for verification.

Following standard skin preparation and the placement of a small keyhole drape, cutaneous anesthesia is carried out. The short 25-gauge needle used for cutaneous anesthesia is left in place in the skin, angled at the expected skin entry angle for the actual biopsy, and a single CT image is obtained at the axial level of the needle (Fig. 9–3). This permits final readjustment of needle entry site and angulation. In most cases, systemic analgesia is unnecessary. If desired, short-acting intravenous or intramuscular analgesia can be given, but these medications are administered only if the patient will not be driving after the procedure.

After a skin nick is made with a pointed scalpel blade, the biopsy needle is inserted. Most commercially available biopsy kits (Fig. 9–4) include a 22-gauge needle, a small ruler for judging depth of insertion, and a syringe for aspiration during biopsy. If the depth of biopsy as

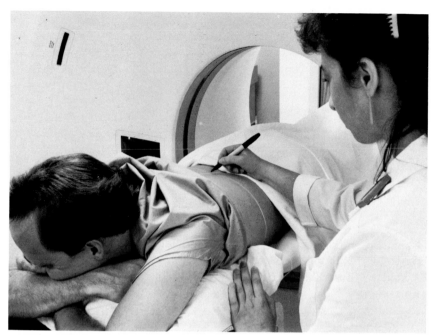

Figure 9–1. Technique of CT-guided biopsy. A technician marks the appropriate CT slice on the skin surface.

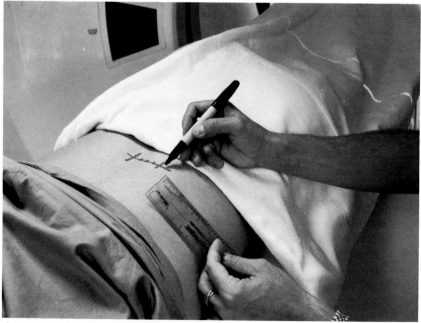

Figure 9–2. Using the spinous process as a midline mark, the entrance for the needle is marked off in centimeter gradations to the side.

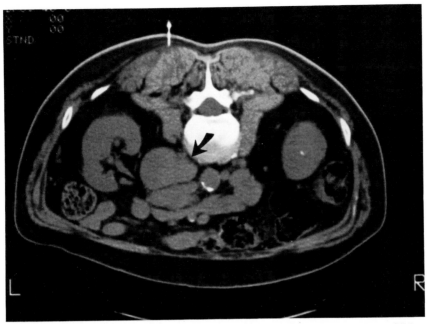

Figure 9–3. A 25-gauge needle for cutaneous anesthesia is left in place, and an additional CT slice is performed. The needle can be seen directed in appropriate angulation toward a left paraspinal mass (arrow).

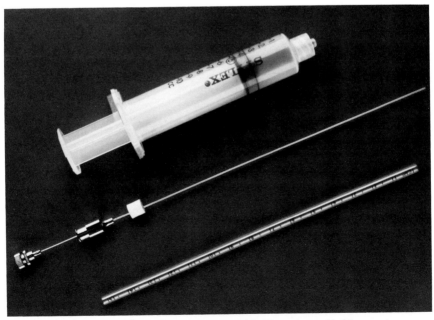

Figure 9–4. A typical commercially available 22-gauge needle biopsy set.

measured from the CT image is deep, it is useful to insert the biopsy needle to partial depth and then obtain a CT image to ascertain the correct route. The needle should be inserted during the same stage of respiration as during the scout CT to ensure proper relationships of organs, even for abdominal biopsies. Each time the patient is scanned during needle placement, a scout view is taken to determine needle tip position, and three contiguous 5-mm-thick images are taken to guarantee that the needle tip is seen. The tip of the needle casts a sharp, low-density artifact (Fig. 9–5).

Once satisfactory needle placement is obtained, the needle stylet is removed, firm suction is applied with a syringe, and the needle is moved in a to-and-fro motion over a range of 5 to 10 mm during suspended respiration. Pressure in the syringe is returned to atmospheric pressure by a gentle release of the plunger, and the needle is withdrawn.

Close coordination with the pathologist is crucial to the success of any needle biopsy procedure. Each institution varies in its methods of tissue handling and fixation, and therefore a discussion with the pathologist prior to a biopsy will ensure the highest diagnostic yield. Ideally,

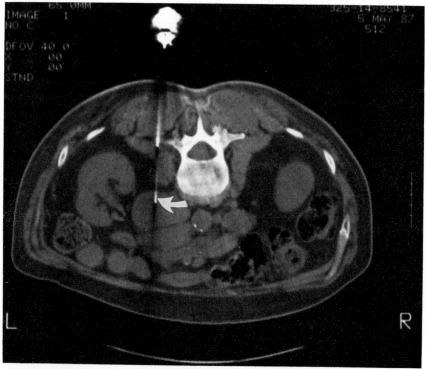

Figure 9–5. The 22-gauge needle is advanced into the left paraspinal mass (arrow), for cytologic sampling.

the pathologist or technologist is present at time of biopsy to prepare slides from the aspirated material. If at all possible, a pathologist can quickly check the sample, within several minutes of the biopsy to guarantee that an adequate diagnostic specimen has been obtained. If inadequate material is seen microscopically, then an additional needle pass can easily be made.

POSTBIOPSY CARE

Close observation for 2 hours after biopsy in the radiology department or in an outpatient recovery area is prudent for most patients undergoing abdominal biopsies. If vital signs are stable, the patient can be discharged to home. If there is a clinical suspicion of hemorrhage or other complication, observation in the hospital can be arranged.

Lung biopsies carry the risk of pneumothorax in approximately 23 to 40% of patients in large series, with 10% of patients requiring placement of a small chest tube with a Heimlich valve for drainage.[3-4] Late pneumothorax is unusual. In a group of 673 patients undergoing transthoracic needle biopsy, 98% of pneumothoraces were detected either on an immediate postbiopsy chest radiograph or on a 1-hour postbiopsy film.[4] Only 2% of pneumothoraces were seen first on a 4-hour postbiopsy radiograph, and none of these late pneumothoraces required chest tube drainage. Therefore, if a 1-hour postbiopsy chest roentgenogram shows no pneumothorax, the patient can be discharged to home. If there is a small pneumothorax (20%) and the patient is asymptomatic, a follow-up film 4 hours after biopsy can be obtained to assure stability prior to discharge. If a chest tube is placed for the treatment of a pneumothorax, many physicians admit the patient to the hospital for overnight observation, although some centers manage these patients as outpatients.[3]

CONCLUSION

Outpatient CT-guided percutaneous biopsy techniques offer a safe and high-yield procedure for the diagnosis of a variety of lesions, with a low complication rate. CT-guided needle aspiration is a straightforward procedure, although often more time-consuming than ultrasonography or fluoroscopy. Close cooperation between the diagnostic radiologist, referring clinician, and pathologist is crucial. Patient acceptance of outpatient biopsy procedures is excellent.

References

1. Smith EH: The hazards of fine-needle aspiration biopsy. Ultrasound Med Biol 10:629, 634, 1984.
2. Bernardino ME: Percutaneous biopsy. AJR 142:41–45, 1984.
3. Stevens CM, Jackman RJ: Outpatient needle biopsy of the lung: Its safety and utility. Radiology 151:301–304, 1984.
4. Perimutt LM, Braun SD, Newman GE, et al: Timing of chest film follow-up after transthoracic needle aspiration. AJR 146:1049–1050, 1986.

Index

Note: Page numbers in *italics* refer to illustrations; page numbers followed by (t) refer to tables.